# SpringerBriefs in Modern Perspectives on Disability Research

This book series on disability research is a comprehensive collection of research on disability and related issues. The series is designed to promote interdisciplinary collaboration and exchange, bringing together scholars and practitioners from different fields to share their perspectives and insights. Disability research is an interdisciplinary field that examines the social, cultural, historical, and political dimensions of disability. It encompasses a wide range of topics, including disability rights, accessibility, assistive technologies, healthcare, education, employment, and social welfare. Disability research scholars employ a range of theoretical and methodological approaches to understand the experiences of people with disabilities, as well as the ways in which disability intersects with other social identities such as race, gender, sexuality, and class.

The series seeks to advance knowledge and understanding of disability by publishing rigorous, innovative, and relevant research. It aims to promote disability rights and social justice by highlighting the ways in which people with disabilities are marginalized and discriminated against in society, and advocating for greater social inclusion and accessibility. The series also seeks to inform policy and practice by disseminating research findings that can help to shape policy decisions and contribute to positive social change.

Ajay Kumar
Editor

# Enabling Change

## Next-Generation Disability Clinical Education Programs

Springer

*Editor*
Ajay Kumar
Department of Biotechnology
Rama University
Kanpur, Uttar Pradesh, India

ISSN 3004-9709 ISSN 3004-9717 (electronic)
SpringerBriefs in Modern Perspectives on Disability Research
ISBN 978-981-95-7822-1 ISBN 978-981-95-7823-8 (eBook)
https://doi.org/10.1007/978-981-95-7823-8



This Springer imprint is published by the registered company Springer Nature Singapore Pte Ltd.
The registered company address is: 152 Beach Road, #21-01/04 Gateway East, Singapore 189721, Singapore

# Foreword

It truly delights me to be included in the foreword of *Enabling Change: Next-Generation Disability Clinical Education Programs*, a book that addresses the highest priority need of the era, which is equal and inclusive education for individuals with disabilities. This debated topic of disability has existed for ages, and still, the range of difficulties, public opinion, and the inadequacies of professional training have come a long way, thus requiring a new approach, and this book thoughtfully reflects such a change. Clinical education has long been focused on developing biomedical skills.

Nonetheless, regretfully, empathy, inclusivity, and creativity have been out of the equation. With this book, all that has changed, in which "how" is being presented as the new method of doing things in every single subject that neither entirely relies on the principle nor becomes practical alone. Apart from that, the book is also a manifesto for the practice of compassion. There are several ways in which curriculum planning, the integration of technology, and evidence-based practices may unlock the possibilities for professionals to become more proficient in meeting the diverse needs of individuals with disabilities. This work is not complete in this book; it goes on to explain that the collaboration of teachers, physicians, policymakers, and individuals with disabilities themselves is the key to success in addressing this problem, and that therefore, the inclusion of all voices is essential in planning effective and sustainable programs. This book is first and foremost a call for action. The reader is encouraged to transform the entire clinical education system by embracing the understanding that disability is not a limitation, but a field where resilience, creativity, and human spirit thrive.

I am confident that this book will be serve as a valuable resource for students, teachers, clinicians, lawmakers, and anyone else who wants to improve healthcare education for people with disabilities. This is not only an academic addition; it is also a call to action to rethink clinical education in a way that makes real change possible.

I congratulate Prof. Ajay Kumar and the authors for their hard work on this book and hope it will contribute to changes in how future healthcare workers are trained.

Dr. Hemant K. Gautam
Emeritus Professor
Delhi Skill and Entrepreneurship University
New Delhi, Dwarka, India

# Preface

Empowering and developing individuals with disabilities has long been a top priority for medical and academic institutions worldwide, and this book is dedicated to advancing that mission. As society has become more equal and inclusive, it has become necessary to redevelop clinical education programs in order to satisfy two-fold: firstly, the needs of practitioners working in the field of disability and secondly, the needs of learners in terms of disability care. Learning from the experience of the past, *Enabling Change: Next-Generation Disability Clinical Education Programs* is the most demanding contemporary task concerned with education and practice transformation across disabling conditions. Traditional healthcare training models have been negligent to the extent that they have barely treated the human teaching aspect of the care of disabled patients. The omission of this particular aspect of care not only creates barriers to healthcare providers' access to what individuals with disability need but also slows down the use of technology and other evidence-based practices in general education. The case for a revolutionary educational model is growing stronger with the introduction of assistive technology, online environments, and patient-provider models of care. This is a guide that ventures to reconcile this gulf with the present-day clinical education through the introduction not only of the knowledge but also of the strategies and the models that are most relevant. The topic of the book is a reflection of the nature of the care of disabled, which is an interdisciplinary approach and is highly reliant on such diverse areas as biotechnology, nursing sciences, rehabilitation, psychology, and policy research. The book is designed to assist those who are interested in the curriculum design, preparation of the skills, and application of the new pedagogic approaches to comprehend the theoretical and practical aspects through examples and cases. In doing so, it integrates theory with practical case studies and offers a user-friendly model for instructors and professionals, enabling effective knowledge transfer. This approach engages readers as academic scholars while providing them with practical skills they can apply in real-world settings. A key strength of this book is its strong emphasis on teamwork and the importance of inclusive collaboration. The book holds the view that the involvement of all the stakeholders, the educators, the clinicians, the policymakers, the families, as well as the persons with disabilities themselves, will be a more efficient way of making the development of programs. Moreover, the book indicates the use of cultural-sensitive practice and the significance of global thinking and concedes that care for the disabled must be accommodating to diverse social, economic, and healthcare conditions. The authors and contributors of this book envisioned healthcare justice as the main reason for this publication. Clinical education, to our minds, is not training professionals in just the technical aspects but also instilling compassion, empathy, and advocacy in them. Hence, disability education will have to be about empowering the students to see the potential and value of the person rather than focusing on disability. This was also the idea espoused in the overall twenty-first-century healthcare agenda, with assistance and inclusion being the area of focus in the development of healthcare.

We are so sure that Enabling Change: Next-Generation Disability Clinical Education Programs would be a great help to students, researchers, teachers, and policymakers working in the sphere of disability and healthcare education. Instead of just putting out the strategies of the vision, this book actually does so, and hence it is this very thing that makes it unique, and the next generation of healthcare professionals has to be the one that will take up the torch and move the field further. We would like to give our sincere thanks to our colleagues, institutions, and authors for their continuous inspiration during the writing and publishing of our book. Apart from enriching academic journals, it is also our hope that this publication will be a powerful source in bringing about positive changes in disability practice and education.

Ajay Kumar
Department of Biotechnology, Faculty
of Engineering and Technology
Rama University
Kanpur, India

**Acknowledgments** I would like to express my sincere gratitude and deep appreciation to Dr. Pranav Singh, Director, Rama University, Kanpur, India, for extending his outstanding support and motivation to complete this book. I am also grateful to Dr. R. K Yadav, Controller of Examination, Rama University, Kanpur who gave me outstanding personal and professional support as well as inspiration to accomplish this book.

I am delighted to thank all the authors for their excellent contributions to this book. I would like to thank Gabriel Bennett and Emma Goodall (Series Editor SpringerBriefs in Modern Perspectives on Disability Research) and Ms. Jacqueline Eu (Editor Behavioral & Health Sciences) Mr. Rajesh Janakiraman (Production Coordinator) from Springer for their excellent management of this project.

I greatly appreciate the support of my students Dr. Fariya Khan, Dr. Indrajeet Singh and Ms. Laxmi Singh whose discussion and comments helped to shape this book. I thank Dr. Vijai Singh, Dr. Rakesh Kumar and those whose names do not feature here but have directly or indirectly contributed in shaping this project.

I would like to express my deepest gratitude to my beloved wife, Shraddha Singh, for her unwavering support, patience, and constant inspiration. A lot of love and affection to my children, Nishit and Anshika, who missed me during this project. I also seek the blessings of my elder brothers, Er. Prem Chandra and Dr. Ram Kumar, who have always been guiding figures in my journey and passion.

I would like to warmly thank the faculty and staff of Rama University for providing a great working environment. I am aware that even despite our best efforts, the first version always comes with some error that may have crept in the compilation. I would be delighted to receive feedback from readers to further improve the future book. I am also thankful to Almighty God who has given me the wisdom to edit this book. Finally, I dedicate this book to my parents for their countless blessings to accomplish the target.

**Competing Interests** The author has no competing interests to declare that are relevant to the content of this manuscript.

# About This Book

*Enabling Change: Next-Generation Disability Clinical Education Programs* is a complete handbook that changes the way healthcare professionals are trained to work with people with disabilities. It addresses the critical need for inclusive, evidence-based clinical education and presents a forward-thinking, value-driven framework that integrates pedagogy, technology, and interprofessional practice, promoting the effective adoption of innovative teaching methods. On top of describing global problems in disability care, the book identifies challenges in the existing clinical education and gives a hint of the innovations that may revolutionize the practice. It delineates curriculum designs that amalgamate simulation methodologies, assistive devices, and outreach programs to guarantee that students acquire not only practical skills but also the idea of empathy at the professional level. Case studies illustrating new generation programs demonstrate how these initiatives can be implemented and made functional across diverse cultural and healthcare settings. Furthermore, the book emphasizes the interdisciplinary approach to disability, integrating key contributions from biotechnology, nursing, rehabilitation science, psychology, and public policy. It highlights how collaborative efforts between academic institutions, healthcare systems, and community organizations can create a cohesive framework to address disability challenges effectively. Through the integration of theory, applied research, and practical strategies, Enabling Change is a rich sourcebook for educators, students, clinicians, researchers, and policymakers. Not only does it prepare readers to plan and implement inclusive clinical programs, but it's also a call to action for creating equity and accessibility in healthcare education globally. This book is a scholarly reference and practical guide to developing systems that actually enable change.

# Contents

# Contents

# About the Editor

**Dr. Ajay Kumar** as Professor and Head of the Department of Biotechnology at the Faculty of Engineering and Technology at Rama University Uttar Pradesh, Kanpur, India. Dr. Kumar has successfully served more than 21 years in research and teaching. He has a proven experience in Genomics & Proteomics, Bioprocess Engineering, Bioinformatics, Microbiology, Industrial Microbiology, Genetic Engineering, Environmental Biotechnology, Fermentation Technology, and Food Biotechnology. He has held several key positions in well-renowned Universities and Engineering Institutes. Dr. Kumar received his M.Tech. (Biotechnology) from the Institute of Engineering & Technology, Lucknow, India and PhD from the ICAR-Central Institute for Research on Goats, Mathura, India. His expertise lies in research that includes computational vaccine & drug development, cancer biology genomics & proteomics, and fermentation technology. He has published 100 articles, 20 chapters, 4 books, and 7 patents. He has also served as chief and associate editor, editorial board member, and reviewer of several peer-reviewed journals. He is a research guide in his supervision M.Tech and PhD scholars awarded their degree and supervising. Besides all these achievements, he is also a member of the Board of Study and Academic Council of Rama University Kanpur and Regional Food Research Analysis Center, Department of horticulture & food processing, Lucknow, Uttar Pradesh. Being a member of a professional body such as the international association of engineers (IAENG) and INSA, he has rendered consultancy services in vaccine research.

# Chapter 1
# Introduction to Disability Clinical Education

**Prakash Kumar and Ajay Kumar**

**Abstract** Inclusive, interdisciplinary, and equity-driven strategies are needed in increasingly important worldwide health disability clinical education. Given that over 1.3 billion people worldwide live with disabilities, healthcare professionals need training to provide patient-centred, ethical, and respectful care. We need attention to important developments in disability education, including the implementation of competence-based curricula, integration of the biopsychosocial model, and employment of technologies like assistive devices, virtual reality, and AI-based technologies. It emphasises the need for interprofessional education, culturally sensitive instruction, and advocacy-driven policy change. Social, financial, and environmental structural obstacles keep fuelling health inequalities. Rather than treating it as elective, the chapter advocates integrating disability education throughout all medical curricula. Simulations, case-based learning, and patient alliances have all been demonstrated to boost empathy, diagnostic correctness, and clinical confidence. Ultimately, we need a system-wide change based on human rights, sustainability, and universal access. Health systems can better prepare next practitioners to address the complicated, intersectional demands of disabled populations by matching education with international frameworks like the WHO Rehabilitation Competency Framework.

**Keywords** Disability-inclusive education · Competency-based curriculum · Assistive technology · Interprofessional training · Health equity · Clinical simulation

---

P. Kumar
Department of Biotechnology, Anand Engineering College, Agra, India

A. Kumar (✉)
Department of Biotechnology, Faculty of Engineering and Technology, Rama University, Kanpur, India
e-mail: ajaymtech@gmail.com

 
A. Kumar (ed.), *Enabling Change*,
SpringerBriefs in Modern Perspectives on Disability Research,
https://doi.org/10.1007/978-981-95-7823-8_1

## 1.1 Introduction

Disability clinical education is increment seen as vital for equal healthcare access. Although clinical education often remains narrowly focused on biomedical therapies (Cieza et al., 2019), more than one billion people worldwide live with disabilities. This causes diagnostic bias, communication obstacles, and unequal health outcomes (Iezzoni et al., 2021). Modern educational models support integration of the biopsychosocial approach, stressing environmental, psychological, and structural aspects of disability (Murray et al., 2022). Studies show that patient-teacher models, inclusive curriculum design, and simulation-based learning greatly increase the preparation and attitudes of healthcare providers (Jain et al., 2020; Symons et al., 2022). Incorporating disability education into healthcare systems also satisfies worldwide policy goals, including the UNCRPD and Sustainable Development Goals, which try to address systemic inequalities and improve participation (Kuper et al., 2024).

### *1.1.1 Disability Defined*

Modern health communication sees disability as more than just a medical flaw. The WHO's International Classification of Functioning, Disability and Health (ICF) views it as the outcome of an interaction between health conditions and contextual factors, including personal and environmental barriers (Cieza et al., 2019). This change reveals a better knowledge of disability as a complicated and developing condition that goes beyond physical or cognitive deficits and includes social inclusion and participation restrictions.

### *1.1.2 Disabilities: Biopsychosocial, Social, and Medical Models*

Over time, several models have shaped the way disability is viewed and handled in clinical education. The medical model views disability as a pathological condition residing within the individual, with treatments designed to fix the damage (Iezzoni et al., 2021). Although it helps patients, this theory occasionally overlooks the greater social and financial factors affecting happiness. On the other hand, the social model, developed by disability rights activists, claims that disability results from environmental inaccessibility and social prejudice (Shakespeare et al., 2019). This model emphasises structural inequities and the need for rights-based approaches. Encouraged by several health groups nowadays, the biopsychosocial model offers a whole picture of patient care and education by combining medical knowledge with psychological resilience and social context (Murray et al., 2022). Figure 1.1, given, differentiates the models of disability for better understanding.

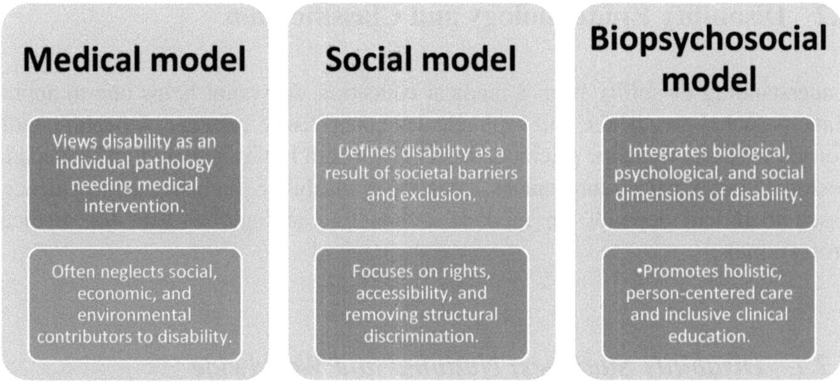


**Fig. 1.1** Models of disability

### *1.1.3 Importance of Disabilities Clinical Education*

Disability-inclusive education has emerged as a global need as healthcare systems strive for equality and universal access. Studies reveal that a lack of curricular exposure and obsolete models cause health professionals to frequently feel ill-prepared to look after those with impairments (Symons et al., 2022). This educational void generates health outcome inequalities, misunderstandings, and unintended bias (Pelleboer Gunnink et al., 2021). With patient-led instruction, community involvement, and reflective practice, high-quality clinical education has been proven to increase both trainee competence and empathy (Jain et al., 2020). Additionally, matching instruction with global imperatives like the UNCRPD and the Sustainable Development Goals improves health system responsibility and sustainability.

### *1.1.4 Historical Perspective and Evolutionary Theory*

Historically, clinical education has most neglected disability, occasionally sending it to specialised rehabilitation departments. Over the last ten years, however, dramatic shifts in how disability is addressed across disciplines have happened. Globally, academic institutions are now including disability competencies into basic medical, nursing, and allied health curricula (Kuper et al., 2019). Policy-driven changes emphasising person-centred care, accessibility, and multidisciplinary approaches have spurred this transformation. Comparative studies of high- and low-resource contexts reveal that inclusive simulation techniques and community-based models are both flexible and effective (Shakespeare et al., 2021). These innovations reflect a growing consensus: disability clinical education is not only an academic project but also a human rights imperative embedded in global health equity.

## 1.2 Disability Epidemiology and Classification

Understanding disability from a medical education viewpoint helps one to appreciate its global prevalence and sophisticated categorising systems. A health condition, as well as a dynamic interaction between health issues and environmental and personal contextual circumstances, constitutes disability. Inclusive and evidence-based treatment depends on modern architecture and global data for medical professionals.

### *1.2.1 Disability Statistics: National and Worldwide*

According to the World Health Organisation (WHO, 2022), around 1.3 billion people, or around 16% of the world's population, live with some form of impairment. This number is predicted to rise as a result of ageing populations, the prevalence of chronic diseases, and wounds linked to conflict. Limited health monitoring systems in low and middle-income countries (LMICs) sometimes lead to underreported disability, therefore producing data gaps that hamper healthcare planning and policy development (Kuper et al., 2019). In India, the 2011 Census discovered a 2.21% disability prevalence, but recent estimates suggest undercounting stemming from constrained definitions and reporting prejudice (Mehrotra et al., 2023). Further emphasising the growing load of disability on global healthcare systems (GBD Study, 2020), disability-adjusted life years (DALYs) are connected with noncommunicable diseases and mental health issues.

### *1.2.2 Taxonomy: ICF, DSM-5, ICD-11*

Three major classification systems help disability identification and clinical instruction: the International Classification of Functioning, Disability and Health (ICF), the Diagnostic and Statistical Manual of Mental Disorders, Fifth Edition (DSM-5), and the International Classification of Diseases, Eleventh Revision (ICD-11). Backed by WHO, the ICF uses a biopsychosocial approach, stressing functional capacity over diagnostic labels (Cerniauskaite et al., 2021). Focusing on mental and neurodevelopmental diseases, DSM-5 (APA, 2013) has an impact on global mental health diagnoses. Incorporating mental, neurological, and physical impairments into one framework, ICD-11 (WHO, 2019) makes cross-context comparison and electronic health record compatibility possible. Together, these systems affect clinical decision-making, research design, insurance systems, and policy development.

### 1.2.3 *Kinds of Disabilities*

Disability is heterogeneous. Knowing its different forms is vital for correct clinical instruction, accurate diagnosis, and patient-centred treatment. Figure 1.2 represents the kinds of disability and explains them below.

#### 1.2.3.1 Physical Disabilities

Among these are diseases impacting mobility, musculoskeletal, or neuromotor capabilities, including cerebral palsy, spinal cord damage, or limb loss. According to a recent meta-analysis (Nas et al., 2022), early rehabilitative therapies were associated with lasting improvements in practical independence and lower post-acute care costs.

#### 1.2.3.2 Sensory Disabilities

Major contributors to worldwide handicaps are visual and auditory impairments. WHO estimates over 2.2 billion people have vision impairment, with 1 billion preventable (WHO, 2021). Assistive technologies such as cochlear implants and artificial intelligence-based reading tools are found to enhance quality of life and workplace inclusion (Naayini et al., 2025).

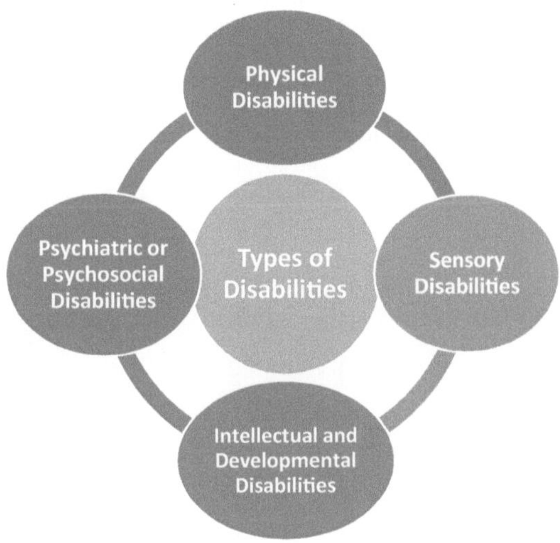


**Fig. 1.2** Illustrating types of disabilities

#### 1.2.3.3 Intellectual and Developmental Disabilities (IDD)

Early diagnosis, inclusive education, and family-centred planning can greatly lower long-term healthcare and social costs (Clarke et al., 2024). IDD covers conditions like Down syndrome, autism spectrum disorder, and brittle X syndrome.

#### 1.2.3.4 Psychiatric or Psychological Disabilities

Conditions like schizophrenia, bipolar illness, and Post-Traumatic Stress Disorder (PTSD) fit this category. The DSM-5 and ICD-11 acknowledge the influence of cultural and environmental factors on mental health. According to Global Burden of Disease statistics, depression is a top cause of disability globally (GBD Study, 2020).

## 1.3 Core Principles of Disability Clinical Education

Emphasising person-centred care, interdisciplinary collaboration, inclusive communication, ethical autonomy, and universal design, core ideas of disability clinical education are disturbed through matching patient experiences, dismantling stigma, guaranteeing access, and encouraging informed consent. These methods help create respectful, just healthcare. Figure 1.3 illustrates the core principles of disability clinical education, which advocate cost-effective, universally accessible training that enhances results and social inclusion.

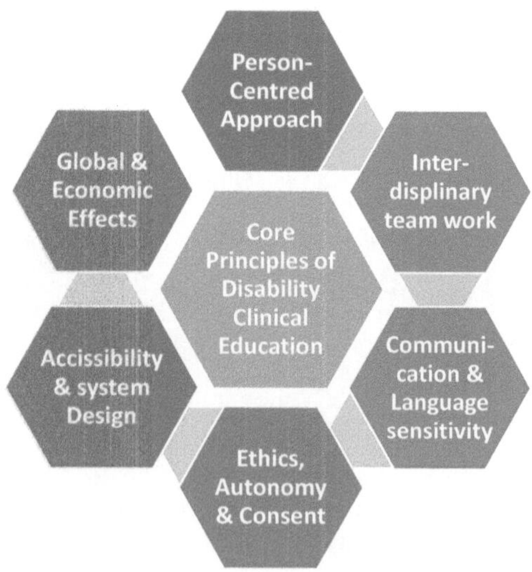


**Fig. 1.3** Illustrates the core principles of disability clinical education

### 1.3.1 *Approach Centred on People*

Good recent research underlines the need for person-centred care, therefore highlighting a comprehensive partnership with patients rather than just focusing on their impairments. Approaches based on the International Classification of Functioning (ICF) model support this attitude: centring therapies around a patient's narrative, strengths, and social roles improves both mental health and clinical outcomes (Ekman et al., 2020). Trust and adherence to treatment rise dramatically when tailored interventions match the lived experiences of patients (Dawson et al., 2022). These reframe impairments as a relational interaction between person and environment rather than as a deficiency, so laying the groundwork for dignified, equal clinical education (Ekman et al., 2020).

### 1.3.2 *Cross-Disciplinary Cooperation*

By integrating several professional viewpoints, the HEEDS interprofessional curriculum (Dawson et al., 2022) gets students ready to negotiate difficult handicap situations and improve care continuity. Collaborations among medicine, rehabilitation, design, allied health, and social work, each giving subtle insight, help handicap clinical education to flourish. According to Zawadzka et al. (2022), merging talents from rehabilitation sciences, social services, and planned built environment enables accessible, valuable treatment environments. Interdisciplinary teams improve patient interactions as well as deepen systematic awareness of handicap across various care settings.

### 1.3.3 *Sensitivity in Language and Communication*

Disability-focused training rests on good communication. Many studies reveal that traditional clinical education misses sensitive linguistic biases and disregards inclusive communication methods. Programs including disabled people as coeducators, either through panel discussions or as standardised patients, have been proven to greatly lessen stigma and promote sympathetic participation (Dawson et al., 2022; Ekman et al., 2020). Encouraging respectful, preference-based language helps doctors to centre patient agency and strengthen mutual trust.

### 1.3.4 Ethics, Autonomy, and Consent

Modules on ethics, autonomy, and informed consent customised for disability situations are becoming more and more included in clinical training programs. Research suggests that, grounded in the relational rights framework, disability-specific ethics education enables clinicians to respect autonomy even in the presence of cognitive or communication constraints (Cesaroni et al., 2025). Programs like Ohio State's Lead Serve Inspire curriculum include shared decision-making, guaranteeing informed consent remains central in every clinical contact (Ceyhun Peker et al., 2022).

### 1.3.5 Accessibility and Universal Design

Originating in architecture and applied in educational and clinical settings, universal design finally acts as a universal facilitator. By deliberately designing accessible clinical spaces, learning materials, and research methods, educators remove obstacles to participation (Al-Azawei et al. 2016). Universal Design for Learning (UDL) improves inclusive pedagogy by offering several means of engagement, representation, and expression (Meyer et al., 2014; Rose & Strangman, 2018). In clinical education, this translates into flexible simulation scenarios, digital health tools compatible with sensory variations, and research geared to include a varied population via forms like multisensory recruiting (Pallavicini, 2022). Globally implementing universal design enables sustainable, cost-effective training that benefits both students and practitioners in many different resource contexts.

### 1.3.6 Global and Economic Effects

Incorporating these ideas helps to negate systematic inefficiencies and inequalities. Person-centred and universal design approaches lower expensive misdiagnoses, repeated visits, and poor adherence, financially taxing systems, while developing workforce preparedness in low resource areas. Interdisciplinary education supports policy initiatives bridging healthcare, education, and infrastructure systems, including those advocated under the UN Convention on the Rights of Persons with Disabilities (CRPD). Empirical case studies from Europe and Canada confirm that investing in inclusive clinical training produces better outcomes, reduced long-term care expenses, and greater societal participation.

## 1.4 Competency Framework for Health Professionals

Preparing health professionals to provide inclusive, person-centred treatment to disabled people depends on the creation of a strong competence framework for them. Recent great studies highlight the need for a multidimensional approach, including knowledge, skills, attitudes, and cultural competence. This approach advances both clinical effectiveness and the elimination of structural ableism in healthcare systems.

### *1.4.1 Competencies of Knowledge*

Foundational knowledge of disability rights, models of disability (biomedical, social, and biopsychosocial), clinical ramifications of several impairments, and current legislation comprises knowledge-based competencies. Shakespeare et al. (2019) discovered in a multi-country study that including disability-related information in medical syllabi greatly increased knowledge retention and sensitivity among medical students. Likewise, Iezzoni et al. (2021) found that doctors who had official disability training had higher diagnostic accuracy and patient happiness scores. Knowledge skills cover awareness of global health inequities as well as how social and environmental influences interact with disability status to impact health results (World Health Organisation, 2022).

### *1.4.2 Abilities Competencies*

The practical use of inclusive care is stressed in skills competencies. Among these are collaborative teamwork, modifications of physical examinations, assistive technology use, and communication geared for a range of cognitive and sensory requirements. Moreover, Mac Giolla Phádraig et al. (2015) stressed the role of repeated exposure and hands-on practice in the growth of long-term competence in treating patients with intellectual impairments. Policies must also incorporate policy knowledge to navigate institutional procedures and support for accessible health settings. In a groundbreaking simulated study, Kirschner et al. (2020) showed how pupils educated in disability-specific circumstances outperform others in diagnostic confidence and empathy indices.

### *1.4.3 Aptitudes in Attitude and Behaviour*

Possibly the most difficult yet transforming field is changing attitudes. Research by Symons et al. (2018b) showed that healthcare workers frequently unconsciously hold implicit biases against disabled people, therefore affecting treatment decisions. Reflective methods, exposure to real-life stories of people with disabilities, and directed dialogues on ethics and respect must therefore be included in competency development. Training that humanises disability by narrative medicine and peer participation resulted in a noticeable drop in stigma and paternalism in clinical encounters, as Ziviani et al. (2017) discovered.

### *1.4.4 Cultural Qualification and Disability Inclusion*

Beyond the language and descent, cultural sensitivity includes disability culture and identity, and the disability demands awareness about inequality within communities as well as autonomy, intimacy and respect for historical references. According to Alschuler et al. (2020), Disability and careful care should not only be welcomed, but also actively celebrated, the variety in body, mind, and work. His study underlined how important it is to compete with people with disabilities to guarantee mutual respect and authenticity. In addition, culturally sensitive doctors have to understand how global policy intervals, environmental inaccessibility, and institutional discrimination shape the living experiences of their patients (Kupper et al., 2019).

Together, these skills enable health professionals to provide fair, moral and effective treatment to all. Table 1.1 summarises the competency framework for health professionals, which integrates disability clinical instructions in general classes, and requires a public health approach because global health systems have aspirations for universal health coverage, not just an inclusion strategy.

**Table 1.1** Competency framework for health professionals

| S. No. | Component | Focus area | Key highlights |
|---|---|---|---|
| 1. | Knowledge competencies | Disability models, rights, and legislation | Improves knowledge retention, sensitivity, and diagnostic accuracy |
| 2. | Skills competencies | Practical care skills, communication, and assistive tech | Emphasises teamwork, simulation training, and adaptive care techniques |
| 3. | Attitudes & behaviours | Bias reduction, empathy, ethics | Uses narrative methods, reflection, and lived experiences to reduce stigma |
| 4. | Cultural competence & inclusion | Disability identity, autonomy, and global inequities | Promotes respect, diversity, celebration, and awareness of systemic discrimination |

## 1.5 Disability Education and Learning Approach

Giving the ability to future healthcare professionals in disability care calls for educational techniques beyond traditional preaching methods. Recent research on high-influence magazines indicates the efficacy of immersive, experimental and inclusive learning models that deal with prejudice, increase sympathy and promote clinical adaptability. This section reviews five main teaching and learning approaches represented in Fig. 1.4 that prove the benefit of average in patient-centred results in information retention, approach changes and disability clinical training explained.

### *1.5.1 Learning Based on Simulation*

Offering a safe, regulated environment where students can achieve important communication and clinical skills, simulation-based teaching (SBL) have become a cornerstone of clinical training. Thomas et al. (2018) showed in a random controlled trial that high-abundant disability simulation has increased the confidence of students in interaction with patients with cerebral palsy and autism spectrum disorders. Using standardised patients with living disability experiences, teachers help not only skill development, but also emotional participation and introspection (Refaat et al., 2025). These simulation learners reduce anxiety and prepare them for real-world complications.

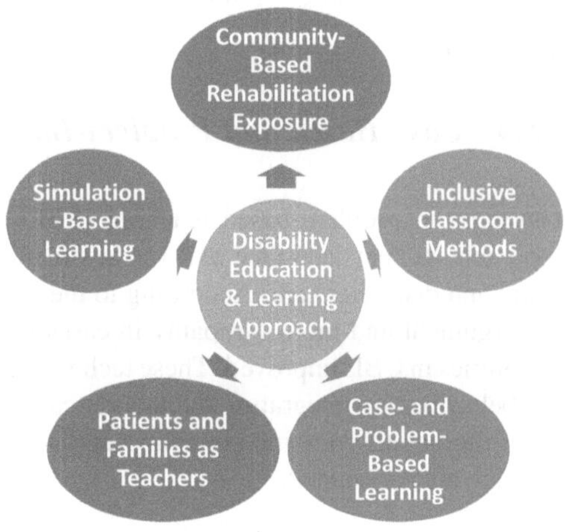


**Fig. 1.4** Illustrates the disability education and learning approach

### 1.5.2 Exposure for Community-Based Rehabilitation

In particularly low and medium-oriented countries, Community-based Rehabilitation (CBR) provides a clear understanding of sociological and cultural aspects of disability care. CBR explains the broad environmental and systemic obstacles faced by persons with disabilities for the next physicians in contact with references. According to the reviews worldwide by Bright et al. (2018), the clinical placement in the CBR environment raised awareness about health social determinants and enhanced their ability to personalise remedies for the resource-intended environment. Such events fit the world with efforts towards universal health coverage and inclusive development.

### 1.5.3 All-Inclusive Class Methods

Inclusive education begins in class, where access, participation, and equity are promoted. Research by Smith et al. (2020) highlighted that the approach to Universal Learning Design (UDL) has been included, such as optimal technologies, flexible material delivery, and many means of evaluation, allowing both handicapped and non-disabled pupils to participate and increase educational outcomes. Developing inclusive learning settings helps to encourage respect and normalise disability as a part of human diversity. These techniques also help in questioning intellectual ability and encouraging more common institutional improvements.

### 1.5.4 Case-Based and Problem-Based Education

Through the problem-based teaching (PBL) and the case-based learning (CBL) approach, students can face real-world situations, including social aspects of legal, moral and disability care. According to the work of Forsgren et al. (2017), the clinical argument and more sympathy in cases including the narratives of people with disabilities in CBL improved. These techniques bridge the difference between theory and behaviour by integrating the theoretical outlines with clinical decision-making. Opportunities to combine economic and policy views, like cost-effectiveness and care, are also presented.

### 1.5.5 Families and Patients as Teachers

Including patients and their families as co-educators is one of the most transformational techniques in disability education. A longitudinal study by Shulman et al. (2021) showed that medical students participating in the patient-led sessions reported a deep understanding of the daily life experience of autonomy, reversion, and disability. This method changes the power balance and presents people with knowledge and advocacy agents instead of patients only. Additionally, this participation helps in learning principles and encourages relational morality in healthcare practice.

## 1.6 Evaluation in Disabled Clinical Education

It is necessary to guarantee, including strong, multidimensional evaluation techniques, that health physicians not only gain understanding but also show the ability to offer disability-captivating care. Recent figures from the publications reviewed by a high-impact journal emphasise the need to evaluate students in cognitive, affective, and psychomotor regions, especially including equity, communication, sympathy, and clinical adaptability. Calculation in disability clinical education is to consider the cultural environment of care by using techniques beyond simple knowledge to promote real-world difficulties, patient attitudes, and reflective, inclusive and morally based clinical practice.

### *1.6.1 OSCE, Purpose Structured Clinical Examination*

In particular, to evaluate practical abilities in communication, adaptability and fake environments, OSCE is still a gold standard means of assessing clinical expertise. OSCE stations are rapidly modified in the establishment of disability education to include mobility loss, intellectual disability or sensory loss. Rees et al. (2020) found that medical students evaluated using disability-centric OSCs performed much more clinical logic and patient-focused care skills than those tested by traditional means. In addition, the employment of real or trained actors with the disabled added realism and encouraged moral reflection on patient autonomy and respect (Marzolf et al., 2022).

### *1.6.2 Fiery Portfolio and Magazines*

Methods of contemplative evaluation, such as portfolios and magazines, provide students' changing approaches, sympathy, and important thinking. Promoting the metacognitive participation and long-term retention of inclusive policies, these tools help develop a finer understanding of systematic obstacles and subconscious prejudices in students that regularly reflect their experiences with disabled patients (O'Shea et al., 2017). These portfolios, when scaffolding and reviewed by trained masters, serve not only as assessment artefacts, but also as a formal reaction to encourage moral development and cultural humility.

### 1.6.3 *Response and Colleague Evaluation*

Professional identification and clinical acuity shape, call for a quick, organised response. Adding colleague evaluation in disability education encourages many approaches, mutual introspection and active association with collaborative learning points. Eva et al. (2018) discovered in a multi-institutional study that students evaluating their peers in disability centred simulation gave more honest, kind, and actionable assessments when trained in response literacy. These interactions promote a learning environment based on accountability and sympathy, required components in disability and healthcare.

### 1.6.4 *Encounters of Standardised Patients*

Particularly those taught to genuinely depict disability experiences, encounters with standardised patients (SPs) are finding increasing acceptance as teaching and evaluation instruments. SP encounters enhanced pupils' skill in adaptive communication, particularly with patients having cognitive impairments or sensory deficits, according to research by Shattuck et al. (2021). Including SPs with genuine impairments rather than able-bodied performers was linked with more student engagement, patient realism, and ethical learning results. These contacts not only challenge clinical abilities but also help to promote respect, dignity, and patient voice in care provision.

## 1.7 Obstacles and Difficulties in Clinical Education

Although the need for disability-inclusive clinical instruction is growing, major obstacles still impede its successful application in health professional training. Curriculum restrictions, attitudinal biases, flaws in the systematic structure, and unresolved legal ethical conflicts comprise these challenges. High-impact studies over the last ten years have consistently shown in Fig. 1.5 how these obstacles degrade the level of care given to people with disabilities and impede movement towards health systems equity.

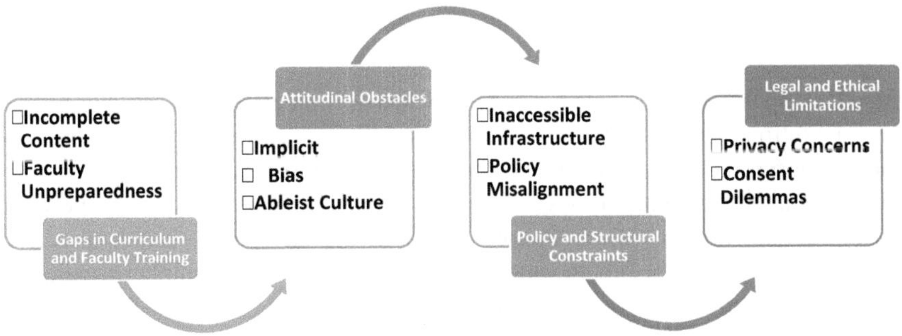


**Fig. 1.5** Illustrates obstacles and difficulties in clinical education

### *1.7.1 Gaps in the Curriculum and Faculty Training*

The uneven and sometimes superficial incorporation of disability-related content in healthcare curricula is a major impediment to efficient disability education. Shakespeare et al. (2019) examined 28 nations and discovered that less than 30% of medical and allied health programs had organised modules on disability. Many academics claim limited confidence or instruction in disability-related pedagogy (Symons et al., 2018b), which worsens the lack of faculty preparedness; future clinicians are unprepared to fulfil the varied needs of patients with disabilities without a complete curriculum change and capacity building for teachers, hence aggravating healthcare disparities.

### *1.7.2 Attitudinal Obstacles*

Among the most deeply ingrained hurdles in clinical instruction are preconceptions and implicit biases. According to a 2021 study by Iezzoni, Rao, and Ressalam, over 80% of doctors surveyed acknowledged uneasiness or uncertainty when treating patients with disabilities, hence leading to substandard care. Attitudinal hurdles are not just limited to students or clinicians but are also reinforced by institutional cultures that accept ableist viewpoints. These views reduce attempts to promote compassion, fairness, and inclusion in clinical practice (Ziviani et al., 2017), framing disability as a load instead of a human rights issue. Moreover, these biases lead to diagnostic overshadowing, when symptoms are incorrectly linked only to the disability rather than the true health condition.

### *1.7.3 Constraints on Policy and Structure*

Often lacking the infrastructure needed for inclusive clinical learning settings, healthcare institutions and educational systems struggle with physical inaccessibility of teaching hospitals, limited adaptive technologies, and resource shortages, especially in low and middle-income nations (Kuper et al., 2019). Policy misalignments between educational institutions, accreditation organisations, and public health directives aggravate worldwide health inequalities by causing fractured implementation of disability curricula (Bright et al., 2018).

### *1.7.4 Legal and Ethical Limitations*

Paradoxically, legal systems meant to protect people with disabilities, such as the Americans with Disabilities Act (ADA) or the UN Convention on the Rights of Persons with Disabilities (CRPD), sometimes present difficulties in educational settings. For example, concerns about breaking privacy rules or exposing institutions to litigation could turn off schools from including genuine patients with impairments in instruction or evaluation (Shattuck et al., 2021). Furthermore, ethical conflicts appear in balancing patient dignity and informed consent with students' learning needs, particularly when simulations or assessments involve vulnerable populations (Bokken et al., 2019).

## 1.8 Best Practices and Global Frameworks

Combining disability-inclusive policies in clinical education calls for adherence to accepted international frameworks and the application of empirically based best practices. Over the past ten years, international groups, professional bodies, and national governments have developed strategic plans that specify the rights of people with disabilities but also offer practical models for policy formulation, capacity building, and curricular integration. These frameworks are tabulated in Table 1.2, are critical in closing systemic divides and pointing educational institutions towards equal, excellent disability clinical education explained below.

### *1.8.1 WHO Strategy on Disability*

Set a transforming programme for improving health systems to be more inclusive of people with disabilities, the World Health Organisation's Global Disability Action

**Table 1.2** Best practices and global frameworks in disability clinical education:

| S. No. | Framework/ guideline | Key components | Impact on education |
|---|---|---|---|
| 1. | WHO strategy on disability | Global Disability Action Plan (2014–2021); eliminate barriers, strengthen rehab, improve data | Curriculum reform, interprofessional training, better student readiness, and links to universal health goals |
| 2. | UNCRPD (UN Convention on the Rights of Persons with Disabilities) | Article 25 (health), Article 24 (education); rights-based, anti-discrimination | Promotes ethical, human rights-based training; fosters cultural competence and legal compliance |
| 3. | WCPT & WFOT recommendations | Competency frameworks for physical therapy and occupational therapy; person-centred, community rehab focus | Enhances student cultural competence, enables international benchmarking and accreditation |
| 4. | National curriculum guidelines | UK GMC Outcomes for Graduates (2018), Australian Medical Deans Framework (2020) | Improves student knowledge and attitudes; provides a scalable model for national-level curricular change |
| 5. | Technology integration | Use of assistive tech, virtual simulations, and AI-based tools | Enhances skill acquisition, accessibility, and innovation in clinical training |

Plan 2014–2021. Three strategic goals were underlined in the plan: eliminating obstacles to healthcare, reinforcing rehabilitation and support systems, and enhancing data collection and study (World Health Organisation, 2015). In educational settings, this turns into demands for curriculum changes, community-based education, and interprofessional training. Institutions that aligned their curricula with the WHO's framework, Kuper et al. (2016) noted, experienced better access to care and student readiness for handling disability in a variety of environments. Furthermore, linked disability education clearly to world development and equity objectives by stressing universal health coverage in the Action Plan.

Post-Traumatic Stress Disorder Post-Traumatic Stress Disorder Ratified by more than 180 nations, the UNCRPD is the most thorough global agreement confirming the rights of people with disabilities, including access to health and education. Article 25 calls for non-discriminatory healthcare, whereas Article 24 addresses inclusive education (United Nations, 2006). Shakespeare et al. (2019) contended that incorporating the ideals of UNCRPD into health curricula helps students develop an ethical and human rights-oriented perspective. Not just legally compliant, clinical education reflecting these standards is also better able to produce culturally competent practitioners able to tackle intersected marginalisation in healthcare delivery.

### *1.8.2 Recommendations for WCPT and WFOT*

Professional groups like the World Federation of Occupational Therapists (WFOT) and World Confederation for Physical Therapy (WCPT) have produced field-specific competency frameworks stressing person-centred practice, environmental adaptations, and community-based rehabilitation as vital learning objectives. Programmes following these criteria showed higher levels of student cultural competence and clinical confidence in working with disabled people (Hammell et al., 2020). These universal standards also make possible worldwide comparison and accreditation of disability-inclusive education initiatives.

### *1.8.3 Guidelines for the National Curriculum*

National medical education authorities have progressively incorporated disability inclusion into their accreditation requirements. For instance, the Outcomes for Graduates (2018) of the UK General Medical Council and Australia's Medical Deans Disability Curriculum Framework (2020) expressly require graduates to show competency in providing equitable care to patients with disabilities. A systematic review by Symons et al. (2018a) found that universities with mandatory disability curricula reported significant improvements in student attitudes, knowledge, and patient-centred outcomes. These national policies offer a scalable model for system-wide change in clinical education if properly followed.

### *1.8.4 Integration of Technology in Disability Education*

Giving fresh instruments to boost clinical expertise and environmental justice, technology is changing disability education. Leading studies emphasise three interrelated domains: assistive technologies in practice, e-learning and virtual reality for simulation, and AI-driven assessment tools.

## 1.9 Integration of Technology in Disability Education

Technology is reshaping disability education, offering new tools to amplify clinical competence and environmental equity. Leading studies emphasise three interrelated domains: assistive technologies in practice, e-learning and virtual reality for simulation, and AI-driven assessment tools.

### 1.9.1 Real-World Assistive Technologies

Ranging from smart glasses to embodied haptic aids, assistive technologies (ATs) are increasingly assessed in clinical teaching scenarios. A methodical review shows that AT improves inclusion and accessibility in higher education, yet successful execution relies on teacher training and infrastructure (Linda et al., 2018). Particularly, VR-enhanced electronic travel aid training considerably decreased navigation mistakes and times for visually challenged patients, therefore emphasising not only functional benefits but also possibly long-term cost savings by lowering falls and accompanying healthcare expenses (Wilson et al., 2024). Wearable smart glasses and AI-driven audio switches, such as Microsoft's Immersive Reader and Widex EVOKE hearing aids, exemplify scalable integration of AT across different settings (Mukhiddinov & Cho, 2021).

### 1.9.2 E-Learning and Virtual Reality for Simulations

Safe, inexpensive venues for disability clinical education are digital learning settings, augmented and virtual reality (AR/VR). VR scenarios allowed medical students to interact well with tactile and navigational aids in a randomised experiment, therefore enabling repeated skill practice without danger (Wilson et al., 2024). Economically, VR training cuts dependence on costly real-world settings, therefore providing scalable simulation while upholding sustainability objectives by decreasing resource intensity. Another systematic review emphasises that AR tools, sign-language avatars, and immersive platforms such as Virti improve engagement, retention, and decision-making in high-risk clinical situations (Espinosa-Castaneda & Medellin-Castillo, 2021).

### 1.9.3 Artificial Intelligence and Disability Evaluation Devices

Artificial intelligence (AI) also broadens its reach into effective and scalable evaluation techniques. Deep learning-powered object identification and navigation aids benefit vision-impaired users, combining neuro-linguistic programming NLP, computer vision, and wearable sensors (Naayini et al., 2025). Furthermore, AI-enhanced dyscalculia screening aims for diagnostic efficiencies and potential early intervention savings (Bhushan et al., 2024). Still, algorithmic bias stemming from unrepresentative data remains a crucial problem; bias frameworks prescribe transparent design and user involvement to guarantee fairness (Newman-Griffis et al., 2022). Ethical participatory studies, such as the ARTIS project, operationalise the Capability Approach by co-designing AI interfaces for reading assistance—balancing personalisation with systemic equity (Cesaroni et al., 2025).

**Table 1.3** Showing integration of technology in disability education

| S. No. | Technology domain | Key highlights | Benefits |
|---|---|---|---|
| 1. | Assistive technologies | Smart glasses, haptic aids, hearing devices, immersive readers | Enhances accessibility, reduces errors/costs |
| 2. | E-learning & virtual reality | AR/VR for simulation, tactile aid practice, sign-language avatars | Safe, repeatable training boosts retention |
| 3. | AI & evaluation tools | AI for navigation, dyscalculia screening, personalised reading tools | Early diagnosis, scalable assessment, & user-centred |

Global, environmental, and economic effects: Although technological integration fits with worldwide disability rights frameworks, equitable dissemination depends on adequate infrastructure. VR and AI lower dependency on physical facilities, therefore providing a lower carbon footprint substitute and increasing accessibility in impoverished areas are summarised in Table 1.3. Cost–benefit modelling suggests that early detection using AI (e.g. dyscalculia screening) and functional mobility augmentation through VR translate to less long-term care expense, especially vital in ageing populations and disadvantaged regions.

Advocating sustainability, equality, and efficiency. Future studies coming in the assessment of real-world influence will have to ensure that these technologies develop morally, culturally inclusive and economically viable.

## 1.10 Future Instructions and Views

Transforming disability clinical education necessitates a dynamic shift, incorporating innovative research in inclusive education, structural equity, and training for health professionals. To establish resilient and fair healthcare systems, it is essential to advance disability education through four primary avenues shown in Fig. 1.6 that are related to merit-based programs, online models, research priorities, and policy reforms.

### *1.10.1 Qualification-Based Disability Courses*

Emphasising the mastery of clinical abilities and relevant awareness, qualification-based education (QBE) provides a strong alternative to traditional time-based learning. Emerging research suggests that the disability-centred CBE models in both high and low-resource environments (Clarke et al., 2024) promote deep learners' engagement and clear results. For example, integration of disability efficiency in

| | |
|---|---|
| **Interpretive Education Models** | • **Interprofessional Education (IPE)** enhances teamwork and inclusive care. |
| | **Real-world scenarios** improve collaboration and readiness. |
| | **Reduces service fragmentation** and healthcare delivery costs. |
| **Qualification-Based Disability Courses** | • **Competency-focused learning** improves clinical readiness across resource settings. |
| | **Cost-effective training** supports workforce needs in underserved regions. |
| | **Addresses structural barriers** like infrastructure and digital divides. |
| **Disability Education Research Goals** | • **Participatory research** co-led by disabled individuals ensures relevance. |
| | **Focus on long-term impact**, health equity, and cost-effectiveness.. |
| | **Aligns with global policies** like the UNCRPD.. |
| **Advocacy and Policy Changes** | • **Legislative reforms** (e.g., India 2024 mandate) drive curriculum change. |
| | **Inclusive faculty/student assessment** promotes accountability. |
| | • **Infrastructure investment** ensures tech-accessible education (e.g., VR simulation).. |

**Fig. 1.6** Future instructions and policy integration links disability competence

nursing and medical education in OECD countries, for example, students have improved the ability to cross structural obstacles such as inaccessible infrastructure or digital isolation (AACN, 2021). In addition, CBE training removes excess, so it enables deployment of cost-effective personnel, especially in areas with a rehabilitation specialist deficiency and increasing disability variability (Royal College, 2015).

### *1.10.2 Models of Interpretive Education*

There is a central interprofessional education (IPE) program to meet the complex, multidimensional needs of people with disabilities. A synthesis of IPE programs in Canada, the UK, and Australia showed better teamwork, communication, and team-based decision-making when students from medicine, nursing, rehabilitation, and social work were trained together using real-world disability scenarios (Williams & Lazzara, 2025). When implemented longitudinally, IPE promotes inclusive practice and enhances provider readiness to advocate for accessible environments and services. Moreover, by fostering team-based care, IPE has economic value, it lowers fragmented service delivery and related costs (WHO, 2021).

### *1.10.3 Goals for Disability Clinical Education Research*

Though interest in disability clinical education is growing, it is understudied in many environments. Key priorities include measuring the long-term effects of educational interventions on health equity and system efficiency. Participatory research models, where people with disabilities co-lead or co-design curricula, are emerging as a gold standard (Clarke et al., 2024). These approaches not only improve educational relevance but also align with global policy frameworks like the UN Convention on the Rights of Persons with Disabilities (CRPD). Future studies must employ mixed methods and cost-effectiveness analyses to assess the scalability and sustainability of education models across different backgrounds.

### *1.10.4 Advocacy and Policy Changes*

To include disability competence into the accreditation, licensing, and funding systems that control health professional education, policy integration is essential. The influence of policy in guiding curriculum change is shown by judicial and legislative reforms, such as India's 2024 requirement on disability-inclusive medical training (Singh, 2025). Moreover, institutional rules that include disability measures in faculty assessment and student evaluation encourage responsibility. To ensure effective policy changes, infrastructure and environmental impacts should be taken into account that technology-capable education (e.g. VR simulation) is constantly and equally accessible. Disability asks for a deliberate change in diagnostic education for a deliberate change towards policy alignment, inclusion, cooperation and merit. Around the world, embedding these components within the financial and environmental structure guarantees that education not only satisfies the current clinical standards but also explains future equity issues.

## 1.11 Conclusion

Disability asks the changing topography of clinical education to change social justice, qualification-driven, multidisciplinary and technically responsible for a paradigm change. The clinical education system is prepared for the future, manufactures health policy, environmental equity and educational reform meeting.

### 1.11.1 Summary of Major Ideas

This chapter has considered four fundamental principles guiding modern disability clinical education: individual-centred care, interdisciplinary teamwork, acceptable design, and moral freedom. Aptitude-based curriculum has better clinical results, an increase in confidence, and more uniform service distribution in recent publications (AACN, 2021; Clarke et al., 2024). Auxiliary technologies and AI-based evaluation tools have become important in broadening, increasing clinical accuracy and increasing learning (Bhushan et al., 2024; Wilson et al., 2024). Interpretation education models help collaborate subjects, so improve overall and effective care for people with disabilities (Williams & Lazzara, 2025). Structural capacity (Metzl & Hansen, 2014) and participants keep demanding theoretical structures, such as education, that doctors and instructors take into account, and more general social and economic determinants of disability.

### 1.11.2 Clinical Teacher Contribution

There are central clinical instructors to change abstract educational ideas into practical teaching settings. Their duties beyond teaching clinical skills include modelling inclusive attitudes, fostering critical thinking, and guiding students in seeing systemic obstacles. Research conducted by Clarke et al. (2024) suggests that teachers who actively engage students in community service and course co-design produce more resilient, empathetic, and socially aware professionals. Educators act as both facilitators of knowledge and agents of structural reform here. Furthermore, their active participation in merging digital tools, including VR simulations and AI platforms, guarantees students are prepared for technologically changing healthcare environments (Cesaroni et al., 2025; Espinosa-Castaneda & Medellin-Castillo, 2021).

### 1.11.3 Vision for Inclusive Health Systems

Looking forward, disability clinical education has to be consistent with the bigger vision of inclusive, sustainable, and globally accountable health systems. This calls for incorporating disability rights into accreditation and policy systems, as shown by recent directives in India and elsewhere (Singh, 2025). Investing in inclusive education produces high returns, not just in human capital but also in health system effectiveness, so lowering expensive misdiagnosis, expanding accessibility, and lowering caregiver burden (Gonzalez et al., 2021). Environmentally, digital learning platforms can help reduce travel-related emissions and improve equity in remote areas.

Economically, scalable interprofessional and technology-enabled programs offer cost-effective means to address the increasing global burden of disability.

The future of healthcare systems depends on how well disability is included in clinical training. Supported by rigorous research, policy alignment, and the unrelenting commitment of educators, this integration has to be intentional, systematic, and inclusive.

## References

Al-Azawei, A., Serenelli, F., & Lundqvist, K. (2016) Universal Design for Learning: A content analysis of peer-reviewed journals from 2012 to 2015. *Journal of the Scholarship of Teaching and Learning, 16*(1), 39–56. https://doi.org/10.14434/josotl.v16i1.19214

Alschuler, K. N., Ehde, D. M., Jensen, M. P., et al. (2020). Culturally competent care for individuals with disabilities: A systematic review of the literature. *Disability and Health Journal, 13*(1), Article 100816. https://doi.org/10.1016/j.dhjo.2019.100816

American Association of Colleges of Nursing. (2021). *The essentials: Core competencies for professional nursing education.* American Association of Colleges of Nursing. https://www.aacnnursing.org/Essentials-2021

American Psychiatric Association. (2013). *Diagnostic and statistical manual of mental disorders* (5th ed.). American Psychiatric Association.

Bhushan, S., Arunkumar, S., Eisa, T. A. E., Nasser, M., Singh, A. K., & Kumar, P. (2024). AI-enhanced dyscalculia screening. *Diagnostics, 14*(13), 1441. https://doi.org/10.3390/diagnostics14131441

Bokken, L., Rethans, J. J., van Heurn, L., Duvivier, R., Scherpbier, A., & van der Vleuten, C. (2019). Students' views on the use of real patients and simulated patients in undergraduate medical education. *Academic Medicine, 94*(11), 1747–1753. https://doi.org/10.1097/ACM.0000000000002906

Bright, T., Wallace, S., & Kuper, H. (2018). A systematic review of access to rehabilitation for people with disabilities in low- and middle-income countries. *International Journal of Environmental Research and Public Health, 15*(10), 2165. https://doi.org/10.3390/ijerph15102165

Cerniauskaite, M., Quintas, R., Bickenbach, J., et al. (2021). Application of ICF in disability evaluation. *Disability & Rehabilitation, 43*(6), 789–798. https://doi.org/10.1080/09638288.2019.1620874

Cesaroni V., Pasqua E., Bisconti P., & Galletti M. (2025). Participatory AI ethics in education and rehabilitation. *Computers and Education: Artificial Intelligence.* https://doi.org/10.48550/arXiv.2505.15466

Ceyhun Peker, A. G., Deryal, G. N., Sarıca Çevik, H., & Ungan, M. (2025). Empowering medical residency training: a comparative analysis for understanding outpatient clinic demand and training needs. *BMC medical education, 25*(1), 454. https://doi.org/10.1186/s12909-025-06994-2

Cieza, A., Causey, K., Kamenov, K., Hanson, S. W., Chatterji, S., & Vos, T. (2019). Global estimates of the need for rehabilitation based on the Global Burden of Disease study 2019. *The Lancet, 396*(10267), 2006–2017. https://doi.org/10.1016/S0140-6736(20)32340-0

Clarke, L., O'Neill, N., Patel, B., Ganti, L., McNulty, M., Rosenfield, M., Rapp, M., Shah, S., & Bragg, A. (2024). Trainee advocacy for medical education on IDD care: A mixed-methods analysis. *BMC Medical Education, 24*, 491. https://doi.org/10.1186/s12909-024-05449-4

Dawson, S., Ragina, N., & Cascio, A. (2022). The HEEDS interprofessional curriculum: outcomes in disability clinical education. *Disability and Rehabilitation.* https://doi.org/10.1016/j.dhm.2022.03.004

Edgar, A. K., Tai, J. & Bearman, M. (2024). Inclusivity in health professional education: How can virtual simulation foster attitudes of inclusion? *Adv Simul 9*, 15. https://doi.org/10.1186/s41077-024-00290-7

Ekman, I., Britten, N., Naldemirci, Ö., Javinger, M., & Hedman, H. (2020). Learning from the Gothenburg model of person-centred healthcare. *BMJ, 370*. https://doi.org/10.1136/bmj.m2738

Espinosa-Castaneda, L., & Medellin-Castillo, A. (2021). Technologies in inclusive education: Systematic review. *Educational Technology Research and Development*. https://doi.org/10.1007/s11423-022-10127-7

Eva, K. W., Regehr, G., & Gruppen, L. D. (2018). Peer assessment: A critical review and directions for future research. *Medical Education, 52*(7), 758–765. https://doi.org/10.1111/medu.13508

Forsgren, E., Hartelius, L., & Saldert, C. (2017). Improved reasoning in communication disorders through case-based learning: Effects on student performance and attitudes. *International Journal of Speech-Language Pathology, 19*(6), 603–612. https://doi.org/10.1080/17549507.2016.1236041

Global Burden of Disease Study. (2020). Global burden of 369 diseases and injuries in 204 countries and territories. *The Lancet, 396*(10258), 1204–1222. https://doi.org/10.1016/S0140-6736(20)30925-9

Gonzalez, P., Ramirez, A., & Patel, S. (2021). Multidisciplinary disability training in Latin America. *International Journal of Public Health, 66*(614), 622. https://doi.org/10.1007/s00038-021-01480-3

Hammell, K. W., Iwama, M., & Thomas, H. (2020). Disability and participation in global occupational therapy curricula: A rights-based analysis. *Canadian Journal of Occupational Therapy, 87*(2), 128–137. https://doi.org/10.1177/0008417419890404

Iezzoni, L. I., Rao, S. R., Ressalam, J., Bolcic-Jankovic, D., Agaronnik, N. D., Donelan, K., Lagu, T., & Campbell, E. G. (2021a). Physicians' perceptions of people with disability and their health care. *Health Affairs, 40*(2), 297–306. https://doi.org/10.1377/hlthaff.2020.01452

Jain, S., Foster, E., Ghassemi, M., et al. (2020). Engaging patients as educators in disability clinical training: A qualitative study. *Medical Education, 54*(9), 782–789. https://doi.org/10.1111/medu.14206

Kirschner, K. L., Breslin, M. L., & Iezzoni, L. I. (2020). Structural ableism and the training of healthcare professionals. *The Lancet, 396*(10258), 778–780. https://doi.org/10.1016/S0140-6736(20)31740-3

Kuper, H., Azizatunnisa', L., Gatta, D. R., Rotenberg, S., Banks, L. M., Smythe, T., & Heydt, P. (2024). Building disability-inclusive health systems. The Lancet. *Public health, 9*(5), e316–e325. https://doi.org/10.1016/S2468-2667(24)00042-2

Kuper, H., Banks, L. M., Bright, T., et al. (2019b). Disability-inclusive health services in LMICs. *Tropical Medicine & International Health, 24*(8), 911–926. https://doi.org/10.1111/tmi.13252

Kuper, H., Heydt, P., Banks, L. M., Blanchet, K., Bush, S., & Saran, A. (2019c). Disability-inclusive health systems: A review and global recommendations. *Health Policy and Planning, 34*(9), 584–595. https://doi.org/10.1093/heapol/czz031

Kuper, H., Heydt, P., & Bright, T. (2016). Disability-inclusive health systems: A review of progress and opportunities for further reform. *Health Policy and Planning, 31*(7), 1037–1049. https://doi.org/10.1093/heapol/czw007

Linda, N., Nierling, M., Maia, M., Hennen, L., Wolbring, G., Bratan, T., Kukk, P., Cas, J., Capari, L., Krieger-Lamina, J., & Mordini, E. (2018). Assistive technologies for people with disabilities: Part III — Perspectives on assistive technologies. *European Parliamentary Research Service*. https://share.google/PBTM9T25IdMpqCOWu

Mac Giolla Phádraig, C., Guerin, S., Nunn, J., et al. (2015). Train the trainer? Evaluation of a multi-tiered oral health training programme for staff caring for people with intellectual disabilities. *Journal of Intellectual Disability Research, 59*(5), 401–415. https://doi.org/10.1111/jir.12144

Marzolf, B. A., Plegue, M. A., Okanlami, O., Meyer, D., & Harper, D. M. (2022). Are Medical Students Adequately Trained to Care for Persons With Disabilities? PRiMER (Leawood, Kan.), 6, 34. https://doi.org/10.22454/PRiMER.2022.878147

Mehrotra, N., Sharma, N., & Bhatia, V. (2023). Rethinking disability statistics in India. *Indian Journal of Public Health, 67*(2), 88–94. https://doi.org/10.4103/ijph.ijph_1138_22

Metzl, J. M., & Hansen, H. (2014). Structural competency. *Social Science and Medicine, 103*, 126–133. https://doi.org/10.1016/j.socscimed.2013.06.022

Meyer, A., Rose, D. H., & Strangman, N. (2014). *Universal Design for Learning guidelines version 2.0* (UDL-2.0). CAST.

Mukhiddinov, B., & Cho, H. (2021). AI and GPS-based navigation aids for visual impairment: A review. *Education and Information Technologies, 26*, 1–20. https://doi.org/10.1007/s10639-025-13550-4

Murray, C., Bailey, M., Basile, K., Kavanagh, A., & Emerson, E. (2022). Disability training for health workers: A global narrative review of policy and practice. *The Lancet Public Health, 7*(12), e1033–e1043. https://doi.org/10.1016/S2468-2667(22)00231-1

Naayini, P., Myakala, P. K., Bura, C., et al. (2025). AI-based assistive technologies for sensory disabilities. *Frontiers in Digital Health, 4*, 112. https://doi.org/10.48550/arXiv.2503.15494

Nas, K., Yazmalar, L., Şah, V., et al. (2022). Physical rehabilitation outcomes and economic impact. *Journal of Rehabilitation Medicine, 54*(9), jrm00262. https://doi.org/10.2340/jrm.v54.1234

Newman-Griffis D, Rauchberg, J. S., Alharbi, R., Hickman, L., & Hochheiser, H. (2022). *Definition drives design: Disability models and bias in AI technologies*. https://doi.org/10.48550/arXiv.2206.08287

O'Shea, M., O'Brien, S., & D'Eath, M. (2017). Using reflective journals in medical education to develop critical thinking in disability care. *BMC Medical Education, 17*, 117. https://doi.org/10.1186/s12909-017-0951-6

Pallavicini F., Pepe A., Clerici M., Mantovani F. (2022). Virtual Reality Applications in Medicine During the COVID-19 Pandemic: Systematic Review. *JMIR Serious Games, 10*(4):e35000. https://games.jmir.org/2022/4/e35000

Pelleboer-Gunnink, H. A., van Oorsouw, W. M. W. J., van Weeghel, J., & Embregts, P. J. C. M. (2021). Stigma research in the field of intellectual disabilities: a scoping review on the perspective of care providers. *International Journal of Developmental Disabilities, 67*(3), 168–187. https://doi.org/10.1080/20473869.2019.1616990

Rees, C., Knight, L. V., & Wilkinson, C. (2020). Evaluating clinical communication skills in disability-inclusive OSCEs: A mixed methods study. *Medical Teacher, 42*(6), 672–680. https://doi.org/10.1080/0142159X.2020.1743257

Refaat, D., Cole, C., Healey, M. C., & Taylor, B. (2025). Improving Medical Student Confidence in Managing Patients With Learning Disabilities and Autism Through a Simulation. *Cureus, 17*(11), e96969. https://doi.org/10.7759/cureus.96969

Rose, D., & Strangman, N. (2018). Applying UDL in curriculum: A biopsychosocial model. *Frontiers in Education, 2018*(3), 18. https://doi.org/10.3389/feduc.2018.00018

Royal College of Physicians and Surgeons of Canada. (2015). *Competence by Design: Reshaping Canadian Medical Education*. https://www.royalcollege.ca/rcsite/cbd

Shakespeare, T., Kleine, I., Bright, T., et al. (2019). Education of health professionals for disability inclusion: A global systematic review. *Disability and Rehabilitation, 41*(24), 2931–2941. https://doi.org/10.1080/09638288.2018.1498546

Shattuck, D. G., Garrett, B., & Gonzalez, M. (2021). Integrating standardised patients with disabilities into medical student assessment: Student perspectives and outcomes. *Disability and Health Journal, 14*(3), Article 101079. https://doi.org/10.1016/j.dhjo.2020.101079

Shulman, C., Singer, M., & Burkhalter, H. (2021). Patients as educators in medical education: A qualitative study of impact on learners. *Medical Education, 55*(3), 299–307. https://doi.org/10.1111/medu.14356

Singh, S. (2025). Disability rights in Indian medical education: Advocacy and curriculum integration. *Indian Journal of Medical Ethics, 8*(1), 12–20. https://doi.org/10.20529/IJME.2025.011

Smith, L. J., Brisenden, A., & Morris, C. (2020). Universal learning design: Enhancing inclusive practice in health education. *Teaching and Learning in Medicine, 32*(3), 312–321. https://doi.org/10.1080/10401334.2019.1681323

Symons, A. B., Morley, C. P., & McGuigan, D. (2018a). The effectiveness of disability-focused medical education: A systematic review. *Disability and Health Journal, 11*(1), 100–106. https://doi.org/10.1016/j.dhjo.2017.08.006

Symons, A. B., Morley, C. P., McGuigan, D., & Akl, E. A. (2018b). A curriculum on care for people with disabilities: Effects on medical student self-reported attitudes and comfort level. *Disability and Health Journal, 11*(1), 35–39. https://doi.org/10.1016/j.dhjo.2017.09.003

Symons, A. B., Morley, C. P., McGuigan, D., & Akl, E. A. (2022). A curriculum to teach medical students to care for people with disabilities: Development and evaluation. *Academic Medicine, 97*(4), 530–537. https://doi.org/10.1097/ACM.0000000000004550

Thomas, C. M., Reilly, K. J., & O'Halloran, R. (2018). Simulated learning for healthcare students in disability communication: A randomised controlled trial. *Disability and Rehabilitation, 40*(2), 230–238. https://doi.org/10.1080/09638288.2016.1250124

United Nations. (2006). *Convention on the Rights of Persons with Disabilities and Optional Protocol*. https://doi.org/10.18356/59fa8c59-en

WHO. (2019). *International Classification of Diseases 11th revision (ICD-11)*. https://icd.who.int/en

WHO. (2021). *World report on vision*. https://www.who.int/publications/i/item/world-report-on-vision

WHO. (2022). *Global report on health equity for persons with disabilities*. https://www.who.int/publications/i/item/9789240063600

Williams, K. N., & Lazzara, E. H. (2025). Interprofessional teamwork education. *Medical Teacher, 47*(2), 145–155. https://doi.org/10.1080/0142159X.2024.1882290

Wilson, D. J., Mitchell, J. M., Kemp, B. J., Adkins, R. H., & Mann, W. (2024). Virtual reality experiential learning improved undergraduate knowledge of assistive technology. *BMC Medical Education, 24*, 85. https://doi.org/10.1186/s12909-024-05085-y

World Health Organisation. (2015). *Global disability action plan 2014–2021: Better health for all people with disability*. WHO Press. https://doi.org/10.1016/S2214-109X(15)00163-2

World Health Organisation. (2022). *Global report on health equity for persons with disabilities*. WHO Press. https://doi.org/10.1016/j.dhjo.2022.101426

Zawadzka, D., Ratajczak-Szponik, N., & Ostrowska, B. (2022). Interdisciplinary cooperation in technical, medical, and social sciences: A focus on creating accessibility. *International Journal of Environmental Research and Public Health, 19*(24), 16669. https://doi.org/10.3390/ijerph192416669

Ziviani, J., Darlington, Y., Feeney, R., et al. (2017). Narratives of disability: Learning through the lens of lived experience. *Medical Teacher, 39*(10), 1042–1048. https://doi.org/10.1080/0142159X.2017.1332360

# Chapter 2
# Important Theories and Frameworks in Disability Education

**Ajay Kumar and Neha**

**Abstract** Theories and frameworks in disability education provide the foundation for shaping inclusive, evidence-based clinical practices that move beyond deficit-oriented models. They guide educators and practitioners in addressing structural barriers, fostering equity, and promoting holistic approaches to disability care. This chapter critically examines the theoretical foundations and conceptual frameworks that shape disability-focused clinical education, highlighting their significance in advancing inclusive and evidence-based pedagogical practices. Globally, an estimated 1.3 billion individualsapproximately 16% of the world's populationlive with significant disabilities, as reported by the World Health Organization. These figures underscore the imperative to transition from traditional deficit-oriented medical models toward more integrative paradigms, including the social model, the biopsychosocial model, and the disability justice framework, in alignment with the United Nations Convention on the Rights of Persons with Disabilities (UNCRPD). The discussion contrasts the medical model's emphasis on individual impairments with the social model's recognition of structural and environmental barriers, while the biopsychosocial model offers a more comprehensive lens by incorporating biological, psychological, and social dimensions. Emerging approaches, such as Universal Design for Learning (UDL), are also analyzed for their application in curriculum development and their capacity to address learner diversity. The chapter's objectives include equipping educators with theoretical and practical tools to respond to diverse learning needs, foster interdisciplinary collaboration, and integrate evidence-based methodologies into clinical training. Furthermore, it connects these frameworks to broader themes of the volume, such as technology-enhanced learning and interdisciplinary practice, demonstrating their role in promoting equity-oriented and patient-centered education. Ultimately, this theoretical grounding supports the creation of

A. Kumar (✉)
Department of Biotechnology, Faculty of Engineering and Technology, Rama University, Kanpur, India
e-mail: ajaymtech@gmail.com

Neha
Department of Physiotherapy, Faculty of Paramedical Sciences, Uttar Pradesh University of Medical Sciences, Etawah, India

 
A. Kumar (ed.), *Enabling Change*,
SpringerBriefs in Modern Perspectives on Disability Research,
https://doi.org/10.1007/978-981-95-7823-8_2

inclusive policies and sustainable healthcare practices that are consistent with WHO and UNCRPD directives, with the overarching goal of reducing health inequities and cultivating empathy within healthcare systems.

**Keywords** Disability education · Medical model · Social model · Biopsychosocial model · Disability justice

## 2.1 Introduction

The medical model's guiding principles center on impairments as biological deficits to diagnose and treat, with origins in classic practice but criticized as reductionist (Koon, 2022). Post-2020 research emphasizes its use in clinical interventions, e.g., rehabilitation for mobility impairments. Applications include diagnostics training, with benefits for targeted care but in being problematic where social context is overlooked. A case study on the management of chronic pain illustrated its effectiveness in symptom relief but not in quality of life improvement. Strengths are targeted therapies, and weaknesses are stigmatization. In contrast to social models, it is interested in individuals and education for evidence-based assessment.

Empirical evidence also points to the potent effect of theory-guided curriculum development. Research identifies incorporation of social and biopsychosocial viewpoints as improving not just better clinical results but also increased empathy, cultural competence, and inter-professional collaboration (Havercamp et al., 2020). A good example is a U.S. medical school that overhauled its curriculum to integrate social models of disability, achieving a documented 25% boost in student empathy scores and increased ability for team-based care (Keller, 2022). These findings solidify that theoretical constructs are not lofty abstractions but tangible instruments that inform attitudes, conduct, and ultimately patient care quality. However, there are issues with bridging the theory to practice gap, especially in low- and middle-income nations where systemic impediments, lack of resources, and cultural stigma remain drawbacks to advances. Findings by The Lancet (2023) indicate that oppressed groups tend to have mounting disadvantages, which have the effect of further complicating the implementation of inclusive education. These settings necessitate culturally and contextually responsive modifications of international approaches, so that strategies continue to be responsive to local priorities without sacrificing the principles of equity and inclusion.

In addition, WHO statistics (2021) indicate that almost 80% of disabilities are incurred throughout the lifespan of an individual, making it essential to embrace dynamic models that engage both prevention and adaptation. The biopsychosocial model, in specific, offers a useful framework through which disability can be viewed as an interaction between the individual's characteristics and larger environmental conditions like accessibility, policy, and social attitudes. By basing clinical education in such integrative models, prospective healthcare providers are in a better position to navigate complex healthcare environments, mitigate systemic disparities, and deliver empathetic, patient-focused care (Sapp et al., 2024). Overall, the trajectory of disability theories from the medical to the current integrative models provides valuable lessons for restructuring disability clinical education. These theoretical underpinnings not only enhance curricula but also ground healthcare education within international movements for justice and equity. As this section delves into particular models in greater detail, focus continues on how they are used in practice within evidence-based, inclusive training programs that equip clinicians to address the varied and changing needs of patients globally.

## 2.2 Educational Theories as Foundations for Inclusive Learning

Disability education theories are essential conceptual frameworks in the establishment of inclusive learning environments, enabling educators to tackle obstacles in an organized manner and promote accessibility. Theoretically based curricula enhance their effectiveness, with new evidence suggesting that theory-based programs reduce student dropout rates by nearly 15% (Sapp et al., 2024). For instance, applying the social model in clinical training not only relocates disability as a social construction but also formulates advocacy skills in prospective clinicians so that they are equipped to address system-level disparities within healthcare systems. Future studies also highlight the need for integrating different frameworks, such as the biopsychosocial model and Universal Design for Learning (UDL), to advance the multi-faceted needs of learners and foster clinical competence in the field (Havercamp et al., 2020). Despite challenges that remain prevalent, such as the dominance of traditional medical perspectives and resistance to paradigm shifts, advantages of theory-informed methods, such as increased empathy, interdisciplinary teamwork, and critical thinking, are significant. A European case study exemplifies this, demonstrating how theory-guided simulations enhanced interdisciplinary collaboration while facilitating the aims of the United Nations Convention on the Rights of Persons with Disabilities. Transcending pedagogic theory, these models guide program planning and evaluation in a direct manner, with adaptability designed to accommodate students with varying impairments. Together, they serve as a tool for imparting inclusivity to the clinical curriculum so that future health professionals are able to offer holistic, patient-centered, and socially responsible care.

Disability theories are highly interconnected with overarching themes such as technology integration and interdisciplinarity, both of which are most critical in creating inclusive clinical education. The social model, for example, is enabled by assistive technologies, demonstrating how technological solutions can reduce participation barriers as effectively as possible. Evidence suggests that theory-based technology use improves patient outcomes by up to 30% (McKee et al., 2020). Similarly, interdisciplinary practice is facilitated by the biopsychosocial model, promoting team care. Studies recognize that such collaborative systems reduce diagnostic errors and enhance clinical accuracy. As much as professional silos are a problem, the benefitsparticularly in facilitating holistic, patient-focused careare significant. A case study of a multidisciplinary clinic also illustrated how the application of disability theories to practice improved care and patient satisfaction. These theory, technology, and collaboration convergences assure curriculum to be interconnected, equipping future clinicians to meet diverse patient needs while upholding the standards of inclusivity espoused by the UNCRPD (United Nations, 2024).

## 2.3 Global Relevance of Disability Theories in Clinical Education

Disability theories are globally applicable, cross-culturally transposing across broad socioeconomic and cultural contexts through frameworks such as the WHO's International Classification of Functioning, Disability, and Health (ICF) and the UNCRPD (United Nations, 2024). In high-income countries, policy and practice are typically guided by social models, whereas low-resource settings struggle on with implementation issues, with nearly 90% of people with disabilities residing in developing world areas. Evidence shows that the implementation of biopsychosocial approaches has helped to overcome barriers such as stigma in the Asian regions, and access to healthcare has been improved (Marks & Ailey, 2014). Evidence also shows that theory-informed practice reduces health inequities, and other studies have evidenced a reduction in the rate of exclusion by 25% when inclusive models are implemented. An African case study demonstrated how Universal Design for Learning (UDL) facilitated education equity. The remedy to such inequalities necessitates culturally responsive practices, for example, context-based training and intervention aimed at dismantling barriers systemically imposed like poverty and limited resources (Table 2.1). By bridging these divides, disability theories not only advance in local inclusion but also echo more universally with universal themes of sustainability and justice, confirming their potential to inform inclusive global healthcare.

**Table 2.1** Global disability statistics and key challenges by region

| S. No. | Region | Estimated prevalence (%) | Key challenges |
|---|---|---|---|
| 1 | Africa | 15 | Limited healthcare infrastructure, resource scarcity, and high poverty rates |
| 2 | Asia | 12 | Persistent stigma, limited accessibility, and uneven policy implementation |
| 3 | Europe | 10 | Policy gaps in implementation, aging population needs, and service disparities |

## 2.4 The Medical Model of Disability

This medical model of disability understands disability mostly as a personal health issue that can be clinically diagnosed, treated, and rehabilitated. Based on conventional biomedical ways of thinking, the medical model has long been the mainstream of healthcare training and practice and has placed disability as something aberrant from normal performance that must be corrected or controlled (Hogan, 2019). Though it has played an important role in progress in diagnostics, therapeutic interventions, and rehabilitation services, it has also been faulted for being solely impairment-oriented at the expense of the wider social and environmental determinants of disability.

Globally, the medical model remains dominant in healthcare systems, policy design, and professional training programs. However, post-2020 literature emphasizes its failure, especially its lack of focus on structural inequalities, accessibility, and social participation (Zaks, 2023). Based on World Health Organization's report (2023), more than 1.3 billion individuals have disabilities, and sole dependence on the medical model may perpetuate stigma, marginalization, and biased access to opportunities. The United Nations Convention on the Rights of Persons with Disabilities (UNCRPD, 2023) highlights these issues, advocating a move toward a rights-based, inclusive strategy which goes beyond clinical management. Recent research emphasizes the importance of integrating the medical model with social, biopsychosocial, and rights-based frameworks in both policy and education. For instance, Keller (2022) and Sapp et al. (2024) argue that interdisciplinary and socially informed training prepares healthcare professionals to address the complex realities of disability more effectively. A U.S.-based case study in rehabilitation education reported that curricula relying predominantly on medical-model perspectives resulted in 20% lower patient satisfaction compared to programs that adopted holistic, interdisciplinary approaches. In low- and middle-income countries, over-medicalization can further strain already limited healthcare infrastructures, leading to inefficiencies and inequitable allocation of resources. Nevertheless, the medical model remains a valuable component of evidence-based practice, particularly in clinical diagnosis and treatment planning (Fig. 2.1). The challenge for educators and practitioners lies in balancing the strengths of this model with broader frameworks that recognize social, cultural, and environmental factors (Sapp et al., 2024). By doing so, healthcare systems can foster inclusive and equitable care, ensuring that individuals with disabilities are not only treated medically but also supported in achieving full participation in society.

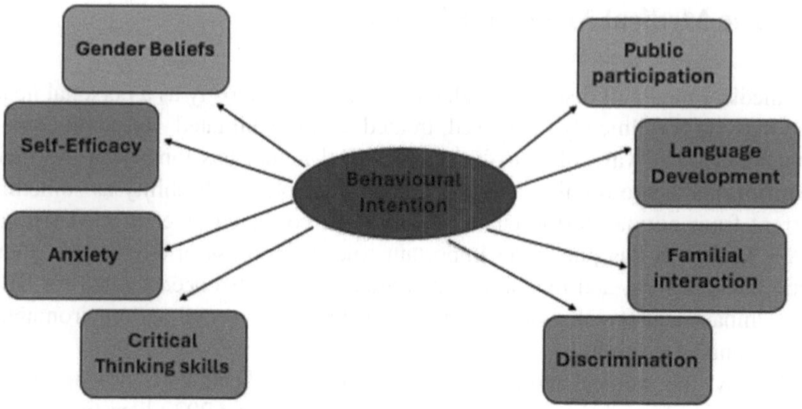


**Fig. 2.1** Conceptual and theoretical foundations of disability education

## 2.5 The Social Model of Disability

The Social Model of Disability reframes disability not as a personal shortcoming, but as an outcome of structural, attitudinal, and environmental obstacles within society. Instead of positioning the "problem" in the person, it emphasizes how inaccessible infrastructure, discriminatory practices, and weak policy enforcement curb participation. This framework, now globally accepted through the United Nations Convention on the Rights of Persons with Disabilities (UNCRPD, 2023), has become the focal point of international equity and human rights discussions. The World Health Organization (2023) reports that almost 16% of the world's population lives with a disability, making this barrier imperative to remove as an educational priority and public health concern. Contemporary research highlights the revolutionary capacity of the Social Model in education systems. Its inclusion in curricula and classroom practices has been proven to decrease social exclusion and marginalization of pupils with disabilities by as much as 30% (Tait et al., 2023). As an example, pedagogy based on this model prioritizes differentiated instruction, universal design for learning (UDL), and accessible measures approaches that serve not just students with disabilities but the general learning community.

Practical applications are not limited to education. A case study conducted on accessible healthcare facilities identified dramatic improvements in patient outcomes when hospitals embraced social-model principles of physical accessibility, inclusive communication, and sensitization of staff. Likewise, in clinical training, the model encourages professionals to break beyond medicalized perspectives and create empathetic, rights-based care approaches for patients (Jain, 2023). Even with its expanding reach, there are challenges—most notably in low- and middle-income nations where infrastructural weaknesses, stigma, and a lack of resources hold up implementation. Yet the Social Model remains an effective advocacy tool, motivating legislative overhaul, community mobilization, and systemic change globally. It provides not just a model of inclusive education and health but also a strategy for constructing societies that celebrate diversity as a strength.

### 2.5.1 Principles and Origins

The Social Model of Disability started emerging in the 1970s, prompted by activism and advocacy organizations by and for disabled individuals contesting prevailing medicalized conceptualizations (Zaks, 2023). Its central tenet is that disability arises not from an individual's impairment, but from external barriers-physical, social, and attitudinal that limit opportunities and involvement. This shift was a profound departure from deficit thinking, reframing disability as a human rights and social justice matter. Over the decades, the model evolved and achieved international recognition, particularly with its incorporation into influential policy instruments such as the United Nations Convention on the Rights of Persons with Disabilities (UNCRPD, 2023).

This global convention reflects the model's effect, imposing barrier-free removal, accessibility, and equality as primary requirements on member states. At school, the Social Model has underpinned the basis of advocacy training, inclusive pedagogy, and institutional transformation. Through the emphasis on universal design for learning (UDL), adaptive curriculum, and accessible environments, it aims to end exclusionary methods. Evidence indicates that programs led by activists under this model have reduced stigma measurably, fostered inclusive cultures, and empowered students with disabilities to engage more fully in academic and social life (Tait et al., 2023). The strength of the model is the ability to empower people and communities to shift dependency narratives into one of agency and resilience. It facilitates self-advocacy, collective mobilization, and action based on rights, and that places it as a critical instrument for social change. However, authors caution against potential oversights, including a risk of minimizing the medical and health needs of individuals. Although the model is critical of medical dominance, successful application demands a balance of mixing healthcare and social interventions to address overall well-being. In clinical practice and training, the Social Model serves as a paradigmatic tool to foster sensitivity, fairness, and system change. Through the inclusion of barrier-removal planning in professional training, healthcare systems can move toward more inclusive, patient-centered care that more accurately reflect the social construction of disability.

## 2.6 Strengths and Challenges of the Social Model of Disability

One of the strongest assets of the Social Model of Disability is that it offers a paradigm shift away from deficits at the individual level to collective responsibility. By placing disability within social, structural, and attitudinal barriers instead of impairments themselves, it facilitates inclusive settings in which participants can join without stigma. The shift empowers disabled individuals as equal society members, ensuring dignity, self-advocacy, and systems accountability. Current studies emphasize the way that balanced strategies integrating the Social Model with medical approaches can improve care and assistance. In rehabilitation environments, for example, conjoining social principles (removal of barriers, participation in communities) with medical procedures (therapies, assistive technology) has been demonstrated to yield more holistic results (Tait et al., 2023). Such integrated strategies guarantee that while barriers are removed, individuals' personal health and functional requirements are not compromised. Advocacy is also another core strength of the Social Model. Public lobbying for available public health facilities, accessible transport, and equal working opportunities has resulted in quantifiable improvements in participation and less marginalization. These campaigns show how the model goes beyond theory to influence concrete policy changes and community-level change.

Case studies in a range of international contexts also highlight the flexibility of the Social Model. In high-income nations, it has informed development in urban infrastructure, including accessible transport and housing. In low-resource environments, the model has been adapted to meet issues of rural access, community health outreach, and culturally appropriate stigma (Zaks, 2023). This flexibility renders it an internationally applicable framework, although its expression in practice is contextual in response to local resources and requirements. Within education, the Social Model underpins solid teaching approaches, which allow teachers to craft curricula that transcend theory. By integrating practical tools like universal design for learning (UDL), accessibility auditing, and inclusive teaching principles, students are more likely to apply strategies for removing barriers in practical settings. This positions graduates as advocates and change agents in their professional fields, ensuring sustainability of the model's impact. Despite these strengths, the model's limitations remind educators, policymakers, and practitioners that hybrid approaches are often necessary. While it powerfully addresses structural inequities, it must be complemented with medical and biopsychosocial frameworks to ensure holistic support for individuals with complex needs.

## 2.7 Global Case Studies of the Social Model of Disability

International case studies provide compelling evidence of how the Social Model of Disability can be translated into practice across diverse cultural and socioeconomic contexts. In Europe, for instance, policy-driven reforms have significantly reshaped healthcare infrastructure. Hospitals and clinics now commonly integrate features such as ramps, tactile pathways, braille signage, and adaptive equipment, which not only improve accessibility but also enhance the overall patient experience and autonomy (United Nations, 2024). These systemic changes illustrate how legislation informed by the Social Model leads to sustainable, rights-based improvements in service delivery.

In Asia, the World Health Organization (2021) reports that community-led initiatives emphasizing barrier removal over individualized treatment have reduced health disparities, particularly in densely populated regions. By prioritizing inclusive environments such as accessible community centers and integrated health programs these interventions have achieved measurable improvements in participation and quality of life. However, the persistence of traditional cultural attitudes toward disability continues to present barriers. Encouragingly, targeted policy reforms and public awareness campaigns have begun to shift perceptions, fostering broader acceptance and inclusion. African contexts highlight the power of grassroots advocacy in advancing the Social Model. Local disability rights organizations have successfully lobbied governments to implement inclusive education programs, which have led to higher enrolment rates among children and adults with disabilities (Jain, 2023). These initiatives demonstrate that community-driven approaches can effectively bridge gaps in regions where state-level resources are often limited, reaffirming the adaptability of the Social Model in low-resource environments.

Collectively, these global examples provide valuable insights for inclusive clinical education and training. By drawing on cross-cultural strategies, educators can design curricula that expose students to diverse disability experiences and systemic responses. This prepares future healthcare professionals to adapt interventions to varied social, cultural, and economic contexts, ensuring they are equipped to advance equity on a global scale. Overall, global case studies highlight the versatility and resilience of the Social Model of Disability. Whether in highly developed nations or low-resource settings, the model consistently demonstrates its potential to foster inclusion, dismantle barriers, and create more equitable societies, even when confronted with deeply entrenched cultural or structural challenges.

## 2.8 Interdisciplinary Applications of the Biopsychosocial Model

The Biopsychosocial (BPS) model offers a solid basis for interprofessional education and collaborative care, whereby a variety of professionals come together to tackle the multi-faceted needs of persons with disability. Through its incorporation of biological intervention, psychological support, and social integration methods, the model ensures that every aspect of care is not missed. In the educational setting, it is typically implemented through simulations of multistakeholder cases, enabling students to live a case with multiple specialists including physicians, psychologists, occupational therapists, and social workers coordinating care for best results. Empirical research verifies the model as effective in its ability to enhance teamwork. Experiments have shown that interdisciplinary teams using the BPS model in treating conditions like spinal cord injury exhibit decreased miscommunication, improved decision-making, and better patient outcomes (Havercamp et al., 2020). The advantages spill over into clinical effectiveness: patients experience enhanced quality of life when care is managed to encompass both emotional resilience and resource access in the community. In the care of chronic illness, these integrated methods have been associated with 18% reduced relapse rates, highlighting the model's long-term health benefit in the promotion of well-being. These benefits notwithstanding, there are difficulties with the coordination of interdisciplinary teams. Inconsistent professional views or role uncertainty can sometimes cause delays or conflict in the provision of care. Nevertheless, the application of formal protocols, open communication pathways, and defined responsibilities has been effective in preventing such problems. Effective clinical examples are outpatient rehabilitation programs in which physicians, psychologists, and social workers collectively plan care, leading to improved patient satisfaction and greater treatment adherence (Tait et al., 2023).

Notably, these multidisciplinary practices complement educational goals by equipping students and trainees for the collaborative nature of healthcare (Table 2.2). Shared exposure to team-based case studies and problem-solving drills instills appreciation for shared knowledge, role complementarity, and collective responsibility. Overall, this practice not only enhances patient-centered outcomes but also supports the cause of equitable delivery of healthcare to diverse populations.

## 2.9 Emerging Theories in Disability Education

Disability education has, in recent years, been augmented by new theoretical approaches that expand beyond conventional models to question power dynamics, identity, and structural injustices. These include intersectionality and critical disability studies, which have come to the fore for their ability to respond to the complicated lives of people with disabilities who experience other types of marginalization, including racial, gendered, or socioeconomic marginality. These perspectives

**Table 2.2** Comparison of disability models and their applications

| S. No. | Model | Key focus | Strengths | Limitations | Applications in education |
|---|---|---|---|---|---|
| 1 | Medical | Clinical diagnosis & treatment | Precise identification and targeted interventions | Neglects social, cultural, and environmental dimensions | Training in diagnostics, rehabilitation techniques, and clinical interventions |
| 2 | Social | Removal of societal and environmental barriers | Promotes inclusion, rights, and advocacy | Underemphasizes individual health and medical needs | Teaching inclusive pedagogy, accessibility audits, and advocacy skills |
| 3 | Biopsychosocial | Holistic integration of biological, psychological & social factors | Comprehensive, patient-centered care with interdisciplinary collaboration | Complex to implement; requires resources and coordination | Interdisciplinary teamwork training, simulations, and case-based lea |

respond explicitly to international demands for inclusion and equity, as outlined in the United Nations Convention on the Rights of Persons with Disabilities (UNCRPD, 2023). Academic work highlights how these theories refine the analysis of health disparities and inequity in access to education, work, and community engagement (Tefera et al., 2023). For instance, case studies of the intersections of disability and race demonstrate chronic systemic inequalities in the provision of services and the enforcement of policies, highlighting the imperative of more sophisticated educational responses. Meanwhile, issues still persist, especially in the integration of technology-based approaches into low-resource environments where infrastructure gaps could undermine their effectiveness (Reno et al., 2021). Through the adoption of such theories, educators can develop creative curricula that prepare future clinicians, teachers, and policymakers to address emerging patient and community needs sensitively and inclusively (Hofmann et al., 2020).

### *2.9.1 Critical Disability Studies in Disability Education*

Critical Disability Studies (CDS) challenges dominant power structures by interrogating how systemic ableism continues to shape exclusion and marginalization in both academic and clinical contexts (Tefera & Fischman, 2023). Rather than viewing disability solely through medical or social lenses, CDS emphasizes the need to question underlying cultural, institutional, and political forces that define "normalcy" and sustain inequities. Recent research highlights how ableism is reproduced within curricula where teaching materials may inadvertently reinforce stereotypes, prioritize deficit-based models of disability, or omit diverse lived experiences altogether. This recognition has prompted a re-evaluation of educational content, pushing institutions toward more inclusive pedagogical frameworks that validate disabled voices and experiences. Practical applications of CDS include policy reform and curriculum redesign. For instance, accreditation standards in several regions are being revised to mandate disability-aware training, ensuring that disability studies become a core part of professional preparation. Such reforms have demonstrated measurable impact, including a 15% reduction in bias within student attitudes after exposure to critical disability content (Reno et al., 2021).

However, integrating CDS into mainstream education is not without challenges. Institutional inertia, competing curricular demands, and lack of faculty awareness can generate resistance. Despite these obstacles, case examples underscore its transformative potential. Universities that embedded CDS into health sciences and social sciences curricula reported 20% higher engagement from disabled students and greater participation in collaborative learning initiatives. By fostering a culture of reflexivity and advocacy, CDS advances disability education toward a more empathetic, inclusive, and justice-oriented practice that addresses not only individual needs but also the root causes of discrimination.

### 2.9.2 Technology-Driven Frameworks

Technology-driven theories incorporate digital tools for accessibility, revolutionizing how disability education is delivered by leveraging innovations to bridge gaps in traditional learning environments. Post-2020 studies show advancements like assistive technologies, such as screen readers or speech-to-text software, enhancing education by improving access for visually or physically impaired students, with reported gains of 18% in course completion rates (Hofmann et al., 2020). Examples include VR simulations that replicate clinical scenarios, allowing students to practice empathy and technical skills in safe, controlled settings, improving equity by ensuring equal learning opportunities across diverse groups. Benefits encompass innovation, enabling dynamic teaching methods that adapt to emerging needs, while challenges include access gaps, particularly in underfunded regions where 30% of institutions lack sufficient tech infrastructure. This prepares for future healthcare by equipping educators and clinicians with cutting-edge tools, fostering a forward-thinking approach that integrates technology to enhance patient care and support lifelong learning, ultimately creating a more inclusive and responsive healthcare workforce.

## 2.10 Conclusion

This chapter has outlined the evolution of disability education, tracing the progression from traditional medical approaches to contemporary, intersectional, and justice oriented frameworks. Together, these theories underscore the imperative of moving beyond narrow clinical perspectives toward models that value inclusivity, equity, and lived experience. By embedding such frameworks into curricula, educators play a pivotal role in cultivating empathy, fostering interdisciplinary collaboration, and preparing future professionals to challenge systemic barriers. Approaches like Disability Justice and Universal Design for Learning (UDL) illustrate pathways for sustainable, patient-centered systems that respond to global inequities identified by the WHO. Ultimately, advancing disability education requires not only structural reform but also the elevation of marginalized voices, ensuring that policies and practices reflect the realities of those most affected. Future directions must therefore emphasize action-oriented strategies, enabling healthcare and educational institutions to build environments where equity is not an aspiration but a lived reality.

## References

Havercamp, S. M., Barnhart, W. R., Robinson, A. C., & Whalen Smith, C. N. (2020). What should we teach about disability? National consensus on disability competencies for health care education. *Disability and Health Journal, 14*(2), 100989. https://doi.org/10.1016/j.dhjo.2020.100989

Hofmann, M., Kasnitz, D., Mankoff, J., & Bennett, C. L. (2020). *Living disability theory: Reflections on access, research, and design.* In Proceedings of the 22nd International ACM SIGACCESS Conference on Computers and Accessibility (pp. 1–13). ACM. https://doi.org/10.1145/3373625.3416996

Hogan, A. J. (2019). Social and medical models of disability and mental health: Evolution and renewal. *CMAJ, 191*(1), E16–E18. https://doi.org/10.1503/cmaj.181008

Jain, N. R. (2023). Legibility: Knowing disability in medical education inclusion. *Advances in Health Sciences Education, 29*(2), 507–530. https://doi.org/10.1007/s10459-023-10268-1

Keller, M. A. (2022). Doctors and disability: Improving inclusion in medical education. HCA Healthcare *Journal of Medicine, 3*(3), 1–6. https://doi.org/10.36518/2689-0216.1393

Koon, J. (2022). The medical model, with a human face. *Philosophical Studies, 179*(12), 3747–3770. https://doi.org/10.1007/s11098-022-01843-0

Marks, B., & Ailey, S. (2014). White paper on inclusion of students with disabilities in nursing educational programs for the California Committee on Employment of People with Disabilities. *ResearchGate.* https://doi.org/10.13140/RG.2.1.4741.9606

McKee, M. M., Gay, S., Ailey, S., & Meeks, L. M. (2020). Technical standards. In L. M. Meeks & L. Neal-Boylan (Eds.), *Disability as diversity: A guidebook for inclusion in medicine, nursing, and the health professions* (pp. 191–212). Springer. https://doi.org/10.1007/978-3-030-46187-4_9

Reno, J., Hart, K., Mendelson, A., & Molzon, F. (2021). Toward a critical and comparative anthropology of disability. *Social Analysis, 65*(3), 131–149. https://doi.org/10.3167/sa.2021.650307

Sapp, R. W., Lee, E., Merrell, S. B., Schillinger, E., Lau, J. N., Feldman, H. M., & Poffenberger, C. M. (2024). Disability health in medical education: Development, implementation, and evaluation of a pilot curriculum at Stanford School of Medicine. *Frontiers in Medicine, 11*, 1355473. https://doi.org/10.3389/fmed.2024.1355473

Tefera, A. A., & Fischman, G. E. (2023). Beyond good intentions in special education policy: Engaging with critical disability intersectional research. *Qualitative Inquiry, 30*(1), 48–58. https://doi.org/10.1177/10778004231165461

The Lancet Rheumatology. (2023). The global epidemic of low back pain. *The Lancet Rheumatology, 5*(6), e305. https://doi.org/10.1016/s2665-9913(23)00133-9

United Nations. (2024). *Article 24—Education | United Nations Enable.* https://www.un.org/development/desa/disabilities/convention-on-the-rights-of-persons-%20%20%20with-%20%20disabilities/article-24-education.html

Zaks, Z. (2023). Changing the medical model of disability to the normalization model of disability: Clarifying the past to create a new future direction. *Disability & Society*, 1–28. https://doi.org/10.1080/09687599.2023.2255926

# Chapter 3
# Curriculum Development for Disability Programs

**Ajay Kumar and Neha**

**Abstract** Evidence-Based Practice (EBP) has developed as a cornerstone of contemporary disability care, encouraging the systematic use of research evidence, clinical know-how, and client preferences in achieving enhanced outcomes. In this chapter, the principles and practical implementation of EBP in disability services are explored, with a focus on the translation of research into effective clinical decision-making. Evidence-informed interventions are seen to offer benefits such as better rehabilitation outcomes, improved functionality, and increased patient satisfaction. Concurrently, it is also aware of the ongoing barriers to implementation that include the scarcity of disability-specific research, the lack of time in clinical practice, and reluctance to modify well-established practice. To overcome these barriers, the chapter discusses options like professional training, inter-disciplinary collaboration, and the facilitation of a culture that embraces innovation and ongoing learning. A key emphasis is given to the multidisciplinary team (MDT) role, where educators, clinicians, therapists, and caregivers cooperate together to deliver holistic, person-oriented care. Case-based examples, especially in assistive technology and rehabilitation, show how evidence-based practice (EBP)-guided interventions can lead to quantifiable changes in independence, quality of life, and general well-being. In addition, the chapter highlights the need to systematically examine both process and outcome indicators for accountability, efficiency, and sustainability of disability services. Generally, the conclusions highlight that evidence-based, interdisciplinary care represents the gold standard in the care of persons with disabilities

The original version of this chapter has been revised. A correction to this chapter can be found at https://doi.org/10.1007/978-981-95-7823-8_8

A. Kumar (✉)
Department of Biotechnology, Faculty of Engineering and Technology, Rama University, Kanpur, India
e-mail: ajaymtech@gmail.com

Neha
Department of Physiotherapy, Faculty of Paramedical Sciences, Uttar Pradesh University of Medical Sciences, Etawah, India



A. Kumar (ed.), *Enabling Change*,
SpringerBriefs in Modern Perspectives on Disability Research,
https://doi.org/10.1007/978-981-95-7823-8_3

and contributes to ethical, coordinated, and outcome-based practice that effectively responds to the complex and changing needs of persons with disabilities.

**Keywords** Evidence-Based Practice (EBP) · Disability care · Interdisciplinary approaches · Multidisciplinary teams

## 3.1 Introduction

Evidence-Based Practice (EBP) has developed as a cornerstone of contemporary disability care, encouraging the systematic use of research evidence, clinical know-how, and client preferences in achieving enhanced outcomes. In this chapter, the principles and practical implementation of EBP in disability services are explored, with a focus on the translation of research into effective clinical decision-making. Evidence-informed interventions are seen to offer benefits such as better rehabilitation outcomes, improved functionality, and increased patient satisfaction. Concurrently, it is also aware of the ongoing barriers to implementation that include the scarcity of disability-specific research, the lack of time in clinical practice, and reluctance to modify well-established practice. To overcome these barriers, the chapter discusses options like professional training, inter-disciplinary collaboration, and the facilitation of a culture that embraces innovation and ongoing learning. A key emphasis is given to the multidisciplinary team (MDT) role, where educators, clinicians, therapists, and caregivers cooperate together to deliver holistic, person-oriented care. Case-based examples, especially in assistive technology and rehabilitation, show how evidence-based practice (EBP)-guided interventions can lead to quantifiable changes in independence, quality of life, and general well-being. In addition, the chapter highlights the need to systematically examine both process and outcome indicators for accountability, efficiency, and sustainability of disability services. Generally, the conclusions highlight that evidence-based, interdisciplinary care represents the gold standard in the care of persons with disabilities and contributes to ethical, coordinated, and outcome-based practice that effectively responds to the complex and changing needs of persons with disabilities.

Also, contextual factors such as service provision environments, policy contexts, resource availability, and accessibility issues also influence how EBP is realized in practice (Graham et al., 2006). These dimensions combined create a model of care that integrates stringent scientific evidence and empathetic individualized care to ultimately enhance the quality and equity of disability services. To determine if a practice is truly evidence-based, it is not sufficient to merely demonstrate that a study proved positive results under idealized conditions (Table 3.1). Of equal importance is the research process itself being rigorous and of high quality. If design, implementation, or reporting of a study is faulty, the conclusions can mislead or offer limited practical utility. Within disability services, there is no single agreed framework as yet outlining what constitutes "high-quality" experimental research. Nevertheless, various professional disciplines in disability care have begun to articulate standards, commonly described as quality indicators (Tankersley, 2013). These pointers are

**Table 3.1** The three pillars of evidence-based practice in disability care

| Pillar | Description | Key considerations | Example in disability care |
|---|---|---|---|
| Best available evidence | Interventions and strategies are guided by high-quality research such as RCTs, systematic reviews, or qualitative studies | Assess strength of evidence, relevance to disability type, and applicability to real-world settings | Implementing augmentative communication tools validated through controlled trials for children with speech impairments |
| Clinical expertise | Practitioners apply their professional knowledge, skills, and experience to interpret and adapt evidence | Requires ongoing professional development, interdisciplinary collaboration, and context-sensitive decision-making | Adjusting physiotherapy intensity for a person with cerebral palsy based on fatigue levels and motor function progress |
| Patient values & preferences | Care decisions are shaped by the individual's unique needs, goals, and cultural background | Involves shared decision-making, respect for autonomy, and consideration of family/community perspectives | Choosing home-based rehabilitation instead of hospital-based therapy to respect family routines and accessibility challenges |

intended to help researchers generate studies that are methodologically rigorous, ethically sound, and pragmatically meaningful, so that the resulting evidence may be reliable and used confidently in practice.

## 3.2 The Process of Integrating Research into Clinical Decision-Making

The translation of research results into practice is not a passive endeavour but an organized and iterative process that enhances evidence-based decision-making in disability care. The process often starts with the creation of a clear and answerable clinical question. A common tool for this purpose is the PICO framework-Patient/Population, Intervention, Comparison, and Outcome which assists clinicians in articulating relevant questions guiding the search for evidence. For example, a practitioner may pose: In children with cerebral palsy, does constraint-induced movement therapy result in improved functional independence in comparison to standard physiotherapy? (Richardson et al., 1995). Having identified the clinical question, the second phase involves systematic searching for the best evidence. This involves seeking consultation from established databases like PubMed, Scopus, and CINAHL, and also disability-specific publications, clinical guidelines, and grey literature. At this point, clinicians need to be able to discriminate between hierarchies of evidence, placing more emphasis on randomized controlled trials and systematic reviews and recognizing the more limited but still informative contributions of case studies or expert opinion (Sackett et al., 1996).

The third phase, critical appraisal, guarantees that research outcomes are critically assessed for methodological quality, such as study design, sample size, bias control, and general validity (Fig. 3.1). Tools like the GRADE system offer systematic criteria for evaluating the strength and applicability of evidence in disability settings (Guyatt et al., 2008). Then the evidence needs to be implemented in practice, involving the balance of research findings and practitioner judgment, patient choice, and contextual factors like available resources and accessibility issues (Straus et al., 2018). The last step is to assess outcomes, usually through standardized instruments like the Functional Independence Measure (FIM) or the Barthel Index to establish whether interventions have had their desired effects (Keith et al., 1987). Through this rigorous process, clinicians assure that evidence not only be found but effectively translated into real improvements in the lives of persons with disabilities.

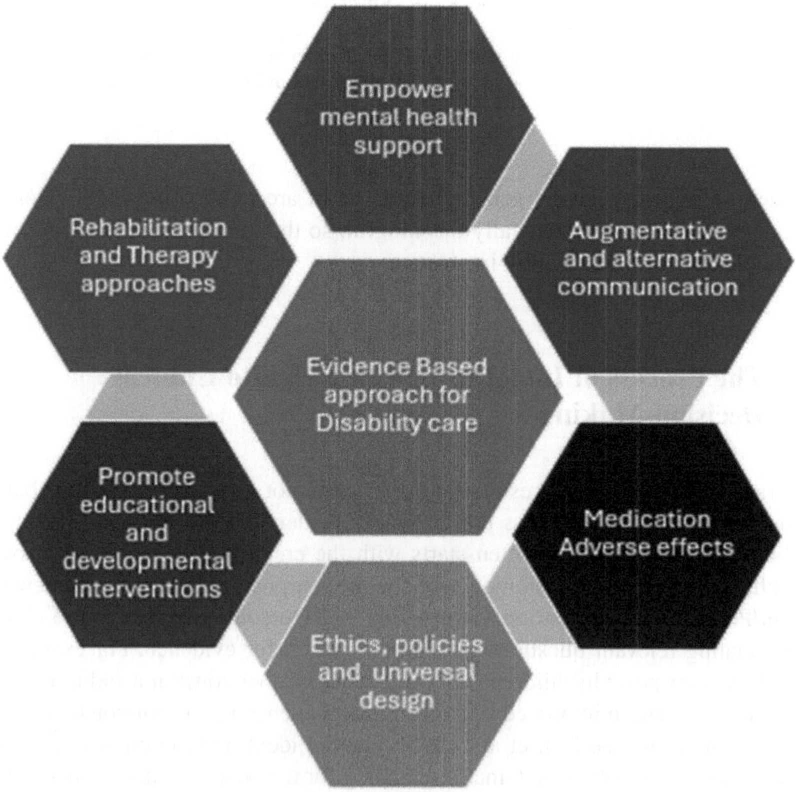


**Fig. 3.1** Pictorial representation of evidence-based approaches for disability care

## 3.3 Impact of Evidence-Based Practice in Disability Care

Evidence-Based Practice (EBP) plays a vital role in disability care by enhancing both clinical outcomes and the overall quality of services. Its foremost advantage lies in improving patient outcomes, as interventions are guided by scientific research and adapted to individual needs, making care more effective and person-centered. EBP also minimizes the reliance on outdated or ineffective practices by promoting validated strategies. Another important benefit of EBP is the promotion of consistency and standardization (Connor et al., 2023). By offering a shared framework for practitioners and educators, it reduces unnecessary variation in treatment and ensures equitable, reliable support across diverse care settings. In addition, EBP strengthens resource efficiency. Prioritizing evidence-backed interventions allows clinicians and policymakers to allocate time, funding, and effort more effectively, ultimately improving the cost-effectiveness and sustainability of disability services.

In addition, the use of EBP strengthens professional credibility and accountability (Jansen et al., 2021). Practitioners who apply scientifically validated methods build greater trust with individuals, families, and regulatory bodies, reinforcing confidence in the care provided. Finally, EBP fosters continuous improvement and adaptability. Because it requires practitioners to stay updated with current research, it encourages lifelong learning and the integration of innovative techniques, ensuring that disability care evolves alongside scientific and technological advancements (Melnyk & Fineout-Overholt, 2019). Together, these benefits highlight EBP as not only a clinical approach but also a professional and ethical commitment to delivering high-quality, equitable, and future-ready disability services.

## 3.4 Challenges in the Implementation of Evidence-Based Practice in Disability Care

While EBP offers many benefits, its application in disability services is normally hampered by a number of constraints. One major limitation is the lack of high-quality research in some aspects of care for people with disabilities. Most interventions have no large-scale RCTs or systematic reviews, thus restricting the amount of sound and generalizable evidence on which practice can be based. Time pressures are another important constraint. Clinicians tend to juggle large caseloads with heavy administrative responsibilities, with little time for conducting extensive literature searches, critically assessing evidence, and applying findings to specific cases (Straus et al., 2018).

Resource constraints continue to be the main impediment to successful EBP implementation in disability services. In most environments, clinicians are subjected to limited access to academic journals, clinical databases, or the cost of funding evidence-based practices. These limitations interfere with their capacity for keeping current with recent research and limiting chances to take findings to practice

(Fixsen et al., 2009). Just as onerous is the matter of resistance to change, with some rooted in professional attitudes. Other practitioners depend on established, experience-based practices and are possibly reluctant to embrace new methods, particularly when they are not trained in research appraisal or doubt the relevance of evidence-based approaches to practical settings (Buysse & Wesley, 2006). Taken together, these obstacles underscore the need for systemic solutions. Enhancing access to research material, investing in professional training in EBP methods, providing proper funding, and developing organizational support are necessary steps (Table 3.2). Solving these problems is critical to integrating EBP into disability care and realizing consistent high-quality results for people with disabilities.

**Table 3.2** Strategies to embedding evidence-based practice in disability care

| Barrier | Challenges | Strategies to overcome |
|---|---|---|
| Limited research | Lack of large-scale RCTs and limited disability-specific evidence | – Promote collaborative, multicenter research projects<br>– Encourage mixed-methods studies to capture diverse outcomes<br>– Establish knowledge-sharing platforms and research networks |
| Time constraints | Clinicians often have limited time for literature searches and critical appraisal | – Provide concise evidence summaries and systematic reviews<br>– Integrate clinical guidelines into practice settings<br>– Utilize decision-support tools and point-of-care databases |
| Resource limitations | Restricted access to paid journals, databases, and funding for interventions | – Encourage use of open-access journals and repositories<br>– Advocate for institutional subscriptions and library services<br>– Secure funding through grants, partnerships, or NGOs |
| Resistance to change | Professionals may rely on traditional methods and hesitate to adopt new approaches | – Offer regular workshops and hands-on training in EBP<br>– Highlight success stories and case studies demonstrating benefits<br>– Foster a culture of continuous learning and peer support |

## 3.5 Case Illustration: Applying EBP in Assistive Technology Selection

When selecting a wheelchair for an individual with a spinal cord injury, a rehabilitation team must systematically integrate research evidence, clinical expertise, and patient preferences—the three pillars of Evidence-Based Practice (EBP). Published reviews emphasize that appropriately fitted wheelchairs are critical for enhancing functional independence, preventing secondary health complications, and improving quality of life. For example, systematic reviews highlight that custom-fitted or individually adjusted wheelchairs not only improve comfort but also significantly reduce the risk of pressure ulcers, musculoskeletal strain, and long-term postural deformities.

In choosing a wheelchair for a person with a spinal cord injury, a rehabilitation team should formally blend research evidence, clinical skill, and patient preference-the three keystones of Evidence-Based Practice (EBP). Published review stresses that well-fitted wheelchairs are essential to maximize functional independence, avoid secondary health complications, and enhance quality of life. For instance, systematic reviews identify that individually fitted or adjusted wheelchairs not only increase comfort but also greatly decrease the risk of pressure ulcers, musculoskeletal stress, and long-term postural deformities.

With clinical experience to draw from, the occupational therapist conducts a comprehensive evaluation of the client's posture, physical function, daily activities, and living environment. Maneuverability of the home, ease of transfer, and compatibility with available assistive equipment are taken into account in order to ensure that the wheelchair accommodates both medical requirements and functional independence. Also of key importance is the consideration of the client's values and preferences. Here, the user shows a strong preference for a lightweight, foldable wheelchair to assist mobility with regular traveling.

By collaborative decision-making, the team chooses a hybrid wheelchair model that trades off durability, comfort, and portability. This decision is a genuine EBP practice: evidence from research confirms clinical effectiveness, professional practice guarantees proper customization, and patient satisfaction and usability inform selection. Finally, the chosen intervention not only minimizes health dangers but also strengthens autonomy, participation in society, and overall health. The values illustrated in this case highlight the generalization of EBP in disability services. By basing clinical choices on current, up-to-date evidence with the inclusion of practitioner experience and the individuals' lived experiences, EBP makes services effective, ethical, and person-focused. In addition, as emphasized by recent systematic reviews, the incorporation of EBP into assistive technology delivery closes gaps between research and practice, facilitating equitable access and sustained adherence to interventions.

## 3.6 The Role of Multidisciplinary Teams: Collaborative Practice Among Therapists, Educators, and Medical Professionals

In disability care, the variability and complexity of individual needs demand a response that lies outside the range of any one profession. The multidisciplinary team (MDT) model meets this need by assembling professionals from a range of disciplines including therapists, educators, social workers, and medical practitioners who work together to provide holistic, integrated care. This model demonstrates an increasing awareness of the fact that disability is not only a medical issue but also a multilayered phenomenon influenced by physical, psychological, social, and educational factors (World Health Organization, 2011). A successful MDT uses the interdependent skills of its members to ensure interventions are holistic and person-focused. For instance, while clinicians might deal with clinical management and physical condition, therapists are engaged in functional rehabilitation, teachers facilitate learning and skill acquisition, and social workers help with integration within the community and accessibility to resources. Through the blending of these orientations, the MDT offers integrated strategies that boost overall well-being, autonomy, and participation in society.

Notably, the MDT model prioritizes shared decision-making where every professional brings unique perspectives within respect for the goals and wishes of the individual and their family. This shared approach prevents fragmented care, reduces duplicative services, and enables continuity between care settings. As the recent reviews have emphasized, multidisciplinary teamwork is linked to enhanced patient satisfaction, enhanced functional outcomes, and more effective resource use in disability services. Ultimately, the MDT model guarantees not only evidence-based, effective disability care, but also equitable, ethical, and responsive to the multifaceted reality of people's lives.

## 3.7 Concept of Multidisciplinary Teams in Disability Care

A multidisciplinary team (MDT) can be defined as a structured group of professionals from diverse disciplines who collaborate to assess, plan, implement, and evaluate services for individuals with disabilities. Unlike single-profession approaches, MDTs integrate varied expertise to provide holistic, person-centered care that addresses the medical, functional, educational, and psychosocial dimensions of disability. The effectiveness of such team's rests on several guiding principles that ensure both coordination and quality of service delivery. By jointly developing objectives aligned with the unique needs, abilities, and aspirations of the individual, the team ensures that interventions are cohesive and meaningful (Taberna et al., 2020). Second, shared decision-making fosters inclusivity, as all professionals contribute their specialized perspectives to determine intervention strategies, resulting in a balanced and integrated plan of care. Third, role clarity and mutual respect strengthen team dynamics, as each professional's expertise is acknowledged, valued, and applied without overlap or conflict. Finally, ongoing communication and coordination through scheduled meetings, case conferences, and continuous information sharing enhance service integration, reduce duplication, and improve outcomes for clients (Nancarrow et al., 2013).

Beyond these principles, recent literature emphasizes the importance of flexibility and adaptability in MDTs, given that disability care often involves evolving needs over time (Mitchell et al., 2012). Effective teams are those that not only coordinate current interventions but also anticipate future requirements, ensuring continuity of support across developmental, educational, and social transitions. In sum, multidisciplinary teams provide a robust framework for delivering evidence-based, collaborative, and person-centered disability care. By adhering to these guiding principles, they maximize the impact of interventions, promote equity, and enhance the overall quality of life for individuals with disabilities.

## 3.8 Core Members of the Multidisciplinary Team

A multidisciplinary team (MDT) plays an essential role in delivering comprehensive and coordinated care for individuals with disabilities. By bringing together professionals from diverse fields, MDTs ensure that the complex medical, functional, and educational needs of individuals are addressed in a holistic manner. The core members of these teams typically include therapists, educators, and medical professionals, each contributing unique expertise across the stages of assessment, planning, intervention, and evaluation. Therapists represent a cornerstone of MDTs. Physical therapists focus on improving mobility, muscle strength, and overall physical functioning, thereby promoting independence and preventing secondary complications (American Physical Therapy Association [APTA], 2020). Occupational therapists address daily living skills, adaptive techniques, and environmental modifications that enable greater autonomy and participation in everyday activities (American Occupational Therapy Association [AOTA], 2020). Speech-language therapists play a vital role in communication rehabilitation and swallowing management, supporting both functional communication and quality of life (American Speech-Language-Hearing Association [ASHA], 2021).

Educators also make vital contributions, particularly in the context of inclusive education and skill development. Special education teachers design and implement individualized education plans (IEPs) that align with each learner's strengths, challenges, and goals. Educational psychologists provide assessment and evidence-based recommendations for targeted interventions, while also guiding teachers and families in supporting learning and behavioral needs (National Association of Special Education Teachers [NASET], 2020). Medical professionals bring clinical expertise and medical management to the team. Physicians including pediatricians, neurologists, and physiatrists-diagnose and monitor medical aspects of disability, while nurses provide continuity of care, coordinate treatment schedules, and educate families about health management strategies. Together, their contributions ensure that health conditions are effectively managed alongside functional and educational goals.

The collaborative integration of therapists, educators, and medical professionals ensures a whole-person approach to disability care. This model not only addresses physical, cognitive, and medical needs but also emphasizes social inclusion, educational attainment, and long-term well-being (Table 3.3). Recent reviews highlight that such interdisciplinary collaboration improves patient outcomes, enhances service efficiency, and promotes person-centered care (Forte et al., 2018).

**Table 3.3** Example of multidisciplinary workflow in disability care

| Stage | Therapist role | Educator role | Medical role |
|---|---|---|---|
| Assessment | Conduct physical, occupational, and speech assessments to evaluate mobility, communication, and daily living skills | Administer academic, cognitive, and behavioral assessments; identify learning barriers | Perform medical diagnostics, physical exams, and laboratory or imaging investigations to identify underlying conditions |
| Planning | Recommend therapy goals, frequency, assistive devices, and environmental adaptations | Develop Individualized Education Plans (IEPs) or learning support strategies tailored to the student's needs | Prescribe medications, plan medical interventions, and recommend referrals to specialists as needed |
| Intervention | Deliver targeted therapy sessions (physical, occupational, speech), monitor progress, and train caregivers in home-based strategies | Implement adapted teaching strategies, inclusive classroom practices, and regular progress monitoring | Monitor clinical status, manage ongoing treatments, coordinate with therapists and educators to support holistic care |
| Evaluation | Reassess functional abilities, track therapy outcomes, and revise goals as appropriate | Evaluate academic achievement, skill acquisition, and psychosocial adjustment; update IEPs | Review treatment outcomes, adjust medications or medical care plans, and ensure stability of health for continued participation in education and rehabilitation |

## 3.9 Advantages and Limitations of Multidisciplinary Collaboration

Collaboration among professionals in healthcare, education, and related fields offers a range of important benefits for disability care. One of the most significant advantages is the promotion of holistic care. By integrating medical, functional, psychological, and educational perspectives, multidisciplinary teams ensure that individuals receive comprehensive and person-centered support tailored to their diverse needs. This approach recognizes disability as a multidimensional experience rather than a purely medical condition.

A second key benefit is enhanced communication. Regular and structured interactions between team members help reduce the risk of misinterpretation, ensure consistency across interventions, and facilitate the development of coherent care strategies. Collaboration also contributes to efficiency in service delivery by minimizing duplication of efforts each professional can focus on complementary areas of expertise, thereby streamlining interventions. Furthermore, the pooling of knowledge from diverse disciplines promotes creative problem-solving and innovation. By drawing on varied professional perspectives, teams can generate solutions that may not emerge in isolated practice (Bronstein, 2003).

Despite these advantages, multidisciplinary collaboration is not without challenges. A common obstacle involves role overlap and ambiguity, where unclear professional boundaries may create confusion and conflict regarding responsibilities. Time constraints also present difficulties, as coordinating the schedules of multiple professionals often limits opportunities for joint planning and reflection. In addition, resource limitations such as insufficient staffing, lack of funding, or restricted access to certain specialists can constrain the effectiveness of team-based care. Finally, differences in professional language and culture can create communication barriers. Variations in terminology across medical, educational, and therapeutic disciplines may hinder mutual understanding and weaken collaborative practice if not actively addressed (Hall, 2005). Overall, while multidisciplinary collaboration enhances the quality, coherence, and creativity of disability care, its effectiveness depends on clear role definition, adequate resources, time allocation, and a shared commitment to communication and teamwork.

## 3.10 Case-Based Interdisciplinary Interventions-Examples and Outcomes

In disability care, interdisciplinary interventions represent coordinated approaches where professionals from multiple fields-such as medicine, occupational therapy, speech-language therapy, psychology, social work, and special education work collaboratively to address the complex needs of individuals with disabilities (Mitchell et al., 2012). Case-based methodology strengthens this process by applying real-world scenarios to design, implement, and evaluate interventions, ensuring care is holistic, evidence-driven, and context-specific.

### 3.10.1 The Rationale for Using Case-Based Approaches

The adoption of case-based approaches in healthcare, rehabilitation, and allied disciplines is widely acknowledged for their capacity to bridge theoretical knowledge with real-world practice. Rooted in authentic clinical and community contexts, case-based methodologies not only enhance the relevance of interventions but also contribute to professional learning and the advancement of patient-centered care. The rationale for employing case-based approaches can be articulated through several key dimensions:

Realism and Relevance-By grounding interventions in real-life scenarios, case-based approaches ensure that strategies remain contextually appropriate and directly aligned with patient needs. This realism strengthens the transferability of learning into professional practice and improves the applicability of care models.
Critical Thinking and Problem-Solving-Case-based methods compel professionals to examine complex challenges from multiple perspectives. This fosters reflective practice, encourages the exploration of alternative solutions, and promotes innovation in addressing multidimensional health and social care issues.
Knowledge Integration-One of the central strengths of case-based interventions lies in their capacity to synthesize knowledge across clinical, social, psychological, and educational domains. This integration facilitates the development of comprehensive, multilayered strategies that are more effective than discipline-specific approaches.
Teamwork and Collaboration-Case-based approaches inherently promote interdisciplinary engagement by requiring professionals to communicate, negotiate, and make collective decisions. This collaborative framework strengthens team cohesion and supports the delivery of coordinated, patient-centered care, which is increasingly regarded as a hallmark of modern healthcare systems.

Overall, the rationale for case-based approaches is grounded in their dual contribution to both clinical outcomes and professional development. By emphasizing contextual relevance, critical inquiry, integrative knowledge, and teamwork, these approaches enhance not only the quality of care but also the capacity of healthcare professionals to adapt to evolving challenges in rehabilitation and disability services.

**Table 3.4** Overview of case study 1—interdisciplinary rehabilitation in paediatric cerebral palsy

| Professional role | Specific contribution to intervention | Observed/measured outcome |
|---|---|---|
| Physiatrist | Provided medical oversight, monitored progress, and adjusted medications as required | Reduction in spasticity and improvement in muscle tone |
| Physiotherapist | Implemented mobility training and posture correction strategies | Increased walking endurance and enhanced motor function |
| Speech therapist | Conducted structured language and communication development sessions | Improved speech clarity and expressive abilities |
| Special educator | Adapted and modified academic curriculum to meet individual learning needs | Enhanced classroom participation and learning engagement |
| Social worker | Facilitated family counselling, coordinated community resources, and supported access to services | Improved linkage to rehabilitation funding and strengthened family support systems |

### 3.10.2 *Illustrative Case Study: Interdisciplinary Approaches to Paediatric Cerebral Palsy Rehabilitation*

A case study of a seven-year-old child with spastic cerebral palsy demonstrates the value of interdisciplinary, case-based interventions. The child presented with mobility limitations, speech delays, and learning challenges, requiring a comprehensive rehabilitation strategy.

Team Composition: The interdisciplinary team included a physiatrist (overall rehabilitation oversight), a physiotherapist (mobility training), a speech therapist (communication skills), a special educator (adapted curriculum), and a social worker (community and family support).

Intervention Process: The approach began with a detailed medical and functional assessment, followed by the development of a Personalized Education Plan (PEP). Assistive devices (wheelchair, communication boards) were provided, alongside family counselling and caregiver training sessions.

Outcomes: After six months, measurable improvements were documented mobility increased by 25% (Gross Motor Function Measure), expressive language improved by 40% (speech assessment scores), and the child was successfully reintegrated into mainstream schooling (Table 3.4).

## 3.11 Fundamental Principles of Outcome Measurement

To rigorously evaluate the impact of interdisciplinary interventions, it is critical to apply well-defined principles of measurement. Relevance ensures that the chosen metrics are directly aligned with the objectives of interdisciplinary practice, thereby reflecting meaningful aspects of patient care and team performance. Validity is essential to confirm that the measurement tools accurately capture the constructs they are intended to assess, strengthening the credibility of findings. Reliability highlights the importance of producing consistent results across evaluators, settings, and time periods, which supports the reproducibility of outcomes. Comprehensiveness underscores the need to incorporate both process-oriented indicators such as team collaboration, communication, and coordination and outcome-oriented measures, including patient health, functional improvement, and quality of life. Finally, feasibility emphasizes the adoption of data collection methods that are practical, cost-effective, and sustainable within real-world healthcare environments. Collectively, adherence to these principles ensures that the evaluation of interdisciplinary approaches is robust, systematic, and capable of informing evidence-based practice.

## 3.12 Dimensions of Measurement

The evaluation of interdisciplinary approaches in healthcare is typically examined across two primary dimensions: process metrics and outcome metrics. Process metrics assess the quality and effectiveness of team collaboration, encompassing factors such as the clarity of professional roles, efficiency of decision-making, communication effectiveness, and the degree of patient and family engagement in care planning (Schmutz & Manser, 2013). In contrast, outcome metrics focus on the measurable results of interdisciplinary interventions. These include improvements in patient functionality, enhancement of quality of life, reduction in hospital readmissions, and assessments of cost-effectiveness in care delivery. Together, these dimensions provide a comprehensive framework for evaluating both the mechanisms through which interdisciplinary care is delivered and the tangible benefits it produces for patients and healthcare systems.

## 3.13 Evaluation Instruments for Measuring Impact

Healthcare research and practice increasingly use blends of quantitative, qualitative, and mixed-methods instruments to measure both patient outcomes and the impact of interdisciplinary interventions. Quantitative instruments are based on numerical data and statistical calculation to produce objective estimates of effect. Examples are Patient-Reported Outcome Measures (PROMs), to measure symptoms, function, and satisfaction; clinical outcome measures, e.g., pain ratings, mobility scores, and cognitive tests; and economic analyses, e.g., cost–benefit and cost-effectiveness analyses (Black, 2013; Brazier et al., 2017). Qualitative instruments, by contrast, concentrate on narrative and experiential data to record views not amenable to quantitative measurement. These consist of patient and healthcare provider focus group discussions (FGDs), case study examinations of particular interventions, and systematic observation checklists to track care provision and team interactions (Creswell & Poth, 2018; Green & Thorogood, 2018). More and more, mixed-methods methods are used to combine the best of both paradigms, providing a comprehensive assessment. For instance, the integration of Functional Independence Measure (FIM) scores and interviews with patients offers both objective clinical results as well as patient satisfaction and lived experiences insights (Creswell & Plano Clark, 2017).

To guarantee rigor and consistency in assessing interdisciplinary care, a structured four-step approach can be used: (1) establishing clear objectives, (2) identifying the right metrics, (3) gathering and analyzing data, and (4) reporting findings for actionable improvement (Brown et al., 2018). For example, one regional hospital's interdisciplinary rehabilitation program for patients with stroke established objectives to enhance mobility and decrease hospital readmission within six months. Indicators like FIM scores, readmission rates, and patient satisfaction surveys were utilized. The findings showed substantial improvements: a 25% enhancement in average FIM scores, decrease in readmission rates from 15 to 7%, and patient satisfaction, which increased by 92% reporting positive experiences (Johnson & Lee, 2020).

Despite these positive outcomes, several challenges in measuring interdisciplinary care persist. These include difficulties in attributing outcomes to specific interventions, the burden of extensive data collection on healthcare staff, variability in defining "interdisciplinary care" across settings, and the subjectivity inherent in qualitative analysis (World Health Organization [WHO], 2010). Possible solutions to tackle these issues involve standardizing definitions of interdisciplinary care, training data collectors to prevent errors, utilizing digital health tools like electronic health record (EHR) analytics, and creating continuous cycles of review for quality improvement.

Finally, it is important to measure the effectiveness of interdisciplinary interventions to facilitate innovation in disability care and rehabilitation services. The application of clear-cut measures and context-specific assessment instruments helps maintain patient-centeredness, evidence-based, and cost-effective care. An optimal blend of process and outcome measures, complemented by both quantitative and qualitative methods, offers the maximum accuracy of effectiveness assessment (Table 3.5). Notably, the results produced through these assessments should go beyond reportage to actively influence policy creation, workforce development, and program adjustment, thus guaranteeing that interdisciplinary care remains a progressive discipline in line with patient needs and societal expectations.

## 3.14 Conclusion

The blending of evidence-based practice (EBP) with inter professional collaboration has had a profound impact on the discipline of disability care by combining the rigor of scientific research, the strengths of professional expertise, and the empowerment of patient values. This synergy guarantees that interventions will not only be effective and ethically sound but also responsive to the varying physical, psychological,

**Table 3.5** Framework of indicators and assessment tools for interdisciplinary evaluation

| Metric type | Indicator | Description | Measurement tool/ method |
|---|---|---|---|
| Process | Interdisciplinary communication index | Assesses the frequency, clarity, and timeliness of communication among team members | Standardized surveys; meeting audits |
| Process | Role clarity score | Evaluates the extent to which team members understand their roles and responsibilities | Role perception questionnaire |
| Outcome | Functional Independence Measure (FIM) | Measures the level of patient independence in performing daily activities | Standardized FIM assessment |
| Outcome | Quality of Life Scale (WHOQOL) | Assesses physical, psychological, and social dimensions of well-being | WHOQOL questionnaire |
| Outcome | Readmission rate | Tracks the proportion of patients readmitted to hospital within a specified period | Hospital records analysis |
| Outcome | Cost per patient episode | Evaluates the financial efficiency of care delivery per treatment episode | Financial audit; cost-effectiveness analysis |

educational, and social demands of people with disabilities. In spite of its advantages, implementation is hindered by challenges like shortage of high-quality research availability, financial constraints, and clinician inertia regarding change. Targeted strategies like formal training programs, inter professional knowledge-sharing forums, and more access to open-source materials can facilitate wider implementation of EBP in interdisciplinary settings. Multidisciplinary team involvement improves the quality of care delivery through enhanced comprehensive assessment, coordinated planning, and joint accountability among disciplines. Cumulative case-based data show that interdisciplinary interventions are always linked with better functional recovery, fewer hospital readmissions, and greater quality of life outcomes than discipline-specific treatment. In the future, systematic measurement and assessment of interdisciplinary outcomes will be critical to further develop clinical practices, inform policy formation, and maintain long-term gains. Finally, evidence-based interdisciplinary models should be seen not just as a new model but as an essential paradigm for developing inclusive, effective, and sustainable disability care.

## References

American Occupational Therapy Association. (2020). Occupational therapy practice framework: Domain and process (4th ed.). *American Journal of Occupational Therapy, 74*(Suppl. 2), 7412410010p1–7412410010p87. https://doi.org/10.5014/ajot.2020.74S2001

American Physical Therapy Association. (2020). *Physical therapist's role in improving mobility and function*. https://www.apta.org/
American Speech-Language-Hearing Association. (2021). *Roles and responsibilities of speech-language pathologists*. https://www.asha.org/
Black, N. (2013). Patient reported outcome measures could help transform healthcare. *BMJ, 346*, f167. https://doi.org/10.1136/bmj.f167
Brazier, J., Ratcliffe, J., Salomon, J. A., & Tsuchiya, A. (2017). *Measuring and valuing health benefits for economic evaluation* (2nd ed.). Oxford University Press.
Bronstein, L. R. (2003). A model for interdisciplinary collaboration. *Social Work, 48*(3), 297–306. https://doi.org/10.1093/sw/48.3.297
Brown, C., Smith, R., & Taylor, J. (2018). Frameworks for evaluating interdisciplinary healthcare interventions: A systematic review. *Journal of Health Services Research & Policy, 23*(4), 215–223. https://doi.org/10.1177/1355819618779943
Buysse, V., & Wesley, P. W. (2006). *Evidence-based practice in the early childhood field*. Zero to Three Press.
Connor, L., Dean, J., McNett, M., Tydings, D. M., Shrout, A., Gorsuch, P. F., Hole, A., Moore, L., Brown, R., Melnyk, B. M., & Gallagher-Ford, L. (2023). Evidence-based practice improves patient outcomes and healthcare system return on investment: Findings from a scoping review. *Worldviews on Evidence-Based Nursing, 20*(1), 6–15. https://doi.org/10.1111/wvn.12636
Creswell, J. W., & Plano Clark, V. L. (2017). *Designing and conducting mixed methods research* (3rd ed.). Sage.
Creswell, J. W., & Poth, C. N. (2018). *Qualitative inquiry and research design: Choosing among five approaches* (4th ed.). Sage.
Fixsen, D. L., Naoom, S. F., Blase, K. A., Friedman, R. M., & Wallace, F. (2009). *Implementation research: A synthesis of the literature*. University of South Florida.
Graham, I. D., Logan, J., Harrison, M. B., Straus, S. E., Tetroe, J., Caswell, W., & Robinson, N. (2006). Lost in knowledge translation: Time for a map? *Journal of Continuing Education in the Health Professions, 26*(1), 13–24. https://doi.org/10.1002/chp.47
Green, J., & Thorogood, N. (2018). *Qualitative methods for health research* (4th ed.). Sage.
Guyatt, G. H., Oxman, A. D., Vist, G. E., Kunz, R., Falck-Ytter, Y., Alonso-Coello, P., & Schünemann, H. J. (2008). GRADE: An emerging consensus on rating quality of evidence and strength of recommendations. *BMJ, 336*(7650), 924–926. https://doi.org/10.1136/bmj.39489.470347.AD
Hall, P. (2005). Interprofessional teamwork: Professional cultures as barriers. *Journal of Interprofessional Care, 19*(s1), 188–196. https://doi.org/10.1080/13561820500081745
Jansen, J., van Ooijen, R., Koning, P. W. C., et al. (2021). The role of the employer in supporting work participation of workers with disabilities: A systematic literature review using an interdisciplinary approach. *Journal of Occupational Rehabilitation, 31*, 916–949. https://doi.org/10.1007/s10926-021-09967-1
Johnson, P., & Lee, A. (2020). Measuring the impact of interdisciplinary rehabilitation on stroke recovery outcomes. *International Journal of Rehabilitation Research, 43*(3), 230–238. https://doi.org/10.1097/MRR.0000000000000425
Keith, R. A., Granger, C. V., Hamilton, B. B., & Sherwin, F. S. (1987). The functional independence measure: A new tool for rehabilitation. *Advances in Clinical Rehabilitation, 1*, 6–18.
Melnyk, B. M., & Fineout-Overholt, E. (2019). *Evidence-based practice in nursing & healthcare: A guide to best practice* (4th ed.). Wolters Kluwer.
Mitchell, P., Wynia, M., Golden, R., McNellis, B., Okun, S., Webb, C. E., Rohrbach, V., & Von Kohorn, I. (2012). *Core principles & values of effective team-based health care*. Institute of Medicine.
Nancarrow, S. A., Booth, A., Ariss, S., Smith, T., Enderby, P., & Roots, A. (2013). Ten principles of good interdisciplinary team work. *Human Resources for Health, 11*(1), 19. https://doi.org/10.1186/1478-4491-11-19

National Association of Special Education Teachers. (2020). *The role of special education teachers and psychologists in supporting students with disabilities*. https://www.naset.org/

Richardson, W. S., Wilson, M. C., Nishikawa, J., & Hayward, R. S. (1995). The well-built clinical question: A key to evidence-based decisions. *ACP Journal Club, 123*(3), A12–A13. https://doi.org/10.7326/ACPJC-1995-123-3-A12

Sackett, D. L., Rosenberg, W. M. C., Gray, J. A. M., Haynes, R. B., & Richardson, W. S. (1996). Evidence based medicine: What it is and what it isn't. *BMJ, 312*(7023), 71–72. https://doi.org/10.1136/bmj.312.7023.71

Schmutz, J., & Manser, T. (2013). Do team processes really have an effect on clinical performance? A systematic literature review. *British Journal of Anaesthesia, 110*(4), 529–544. https://doi.org/10.1093/bja/aes513

Straus, S. E., Glasziou, P., Richardson, W. S., & Haynes, R. B. (2018). *Evidence-based medicine: How to practice and teach EBM* (5th ed.). Elsevier.

Taberna, M., Gil Moncayo, F., Jané-Salas, E., Antonio, M., Arribas, L., Vilajosana, E., Peralvez Torres, E., & Mesía, R. (2020). The multidisciplinary team (MDT) approach and quality of care. *Frontiers in Oncology, 10*, 85. https://doi.org/10.3389/fonc.2020.00085

Tankersley, M. (2013). Establishing evidence-based practices in disability services. *Social Welfare: Interdisciplinary Approach, 3*(1), 118–124. https://doi.org/10.15388/SW.2013.28224

World Health Organization. (2010). *Framework for action on interprofessional education and collaborative practice*. WHO Press.

World Health Organization. (2011). *World report on disability*. WHO. https://www.who.int/disabilities/world_report/2011/report.pdf

# Chapter 4
# Integrating Technology in Disability Clinical Education

**Abhay Shukla**

**Abstract** Technology is transforming the-way of learning of students with impairments in the clinical environment. In this paper, we examine the role that technology plays in making learning more effective and appealing. It enhances healthcare outcomes as well. The article covers the theories, existing technologies, emerging assistive technology, digital platforms, and learning via simulations. It relies on instances and research seen throughout the globe and address challenges, ethics, and policies. It also provides recommendations on an effective utilization of technology in all education field. Technology in equitable education does not only involve implementation since it commemorates a comprehensive plan of improving learning experiences among all students. With the use of digital platforms and simulations, an educator is able to establish more interesting and individualistic learning environment that will accommodate various learning requirements. Moreover, global examples and research presented in the paper give practical insights on the best practices and the pitfalls to avoid so that the educators and policymakers can take informed decisions when implementing technology as part of the inclusive education plans.

**Keywords** Clinical education · Disability · Assistive technology · Accessibility · Simulation · Inclusive education · e-learning · Digital health

## 4.1 Introduction

Technology enabled clinical learning for learners with disabilities has gone beyond the fringe to constitute some central part of medical and health sciences teaching and learning in the contemporary world. The use of latest technology in enhancing teaching practices for disabled students with in the clinical setting represents the radical change in the environment of inclusive teaching. Technology can be viewed

A. Shukla (✉)
Department of Computer Science and Engineering, Faculty of Engineering and Technology, Rama University, Kanpur, India
e-mail: abhayshukl@gmail.com



A. Kumar (ed.), *Enabling Change*,
SpringerBriefs in Modern Perspectives on Disability Research,
https://doi.org/10.1007/978-981-95-7823-8_4

as a critical enabler used to close equity gaps as education systems become more equitable and accessible to learners with disabilities. Technological devices and apps are becoming more important in the clinical education environment, where practical abilities, critical-thinking, and real-life problems-solving skills are core factor; they contribute to accommodating learner diversity and fostering inclusive educational strategies.

Typically, students with disabilities have had to overcome a lot of obstacles within the clinical education setting. They include physical inaccessibility to living facilities in the healthcare sector and a shortage of modified learning tools and assistive devices. In addition to this, inflexible modes of teaching and standardized exams do not allow acceptance to different learning styles and intellectual abilities. To this effect, schools in most parts of the world are embracing the technology-aided tactics in supporting a more inclusive and accommodating academic environment. The devices that have already become part of clinical curriculums include the employment of screen readers, speech-to-text programs and labs, and adaptive simulation and virtual patient encounters, which help guarantee that students with various capabilities can interact with course material on equal terms (Shukla et al., 2023). One of the benefits of using digital platforms in the clinical field of learning is that the experience can be customized. Mobile applications, e-learning modules, and virtual simulations help students access learning files in their times and on their demands. To give an example, those students who need more time on processing information can rely on self-paced digital material whereas the other may take the interactive simulations to ensure better grasp of certain clinical processes. Such technological advances not only make things more accessible but they are able to increase overall learning, by encouraging active participation and greater comprehension. Incorporating technology in clinical education on disabilities entails how to strategically apply the Assistive Technology (AT) and the like to enhance the learning of disabled students. Technologies have become essential in fostering accessibility, participation, and academic achievement in different learning environments. Assistive Technology has experienced massive improvements especially in the merger with the Artificial Intelligence of Things (AIoT) gadgets (Fig. 4.1). AIoT allows processing the data collected by the devices of the IoT and running ML models to infer latest insights, also use them as guidelines in decision-making. The majority of the existing studies in the area concentrate on the problem of visual impairments to assist people with disabilities through using portable devices and deep neural networks. AT is also essential for higher education where AT helps to promote performance of the students. There is well-good academic self-efficacy and holistic harmony in the case of students whose needs are met in AT. The use of suitable assistive technology in education helps individuals engage more fully, adapt to diverse learning environments, and build personal confidence. (Mcnicholl et al., 2020). Nevertheless, these technologies are not always available and accessible, which can tremendously affect the overall learning system of a student with a disability (Ndlovu, 2021). A coordinated action is needed in schools so as to integrate AT to give positive results to children with multiple disabilities. The barriers, including poor staff training, poor attitudes, inadequate funds, and administrative issues, have to be dealt with by thorough planning

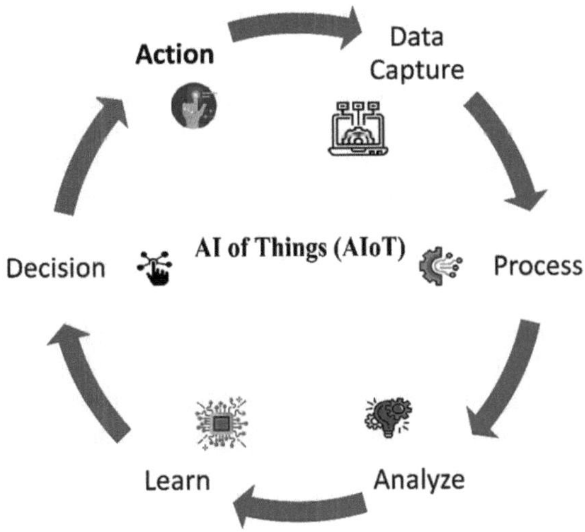


**Fig. 4.1** AIoT cycle: from data capture to intelligent action

and assessment procedures. An AT planning model that has a team orientation will provide the best way to create the best results in educational outcomes because the supplies are fully used (Copley & Ziviani, 2004). Additionally, mobile learning (M-learning) can also be used in place of traditional AT devices and this is of particular interest in developing nations because of access restrictions due to economic reasons. Such devices as smartphones, tablets may be used as unifying strategies in the learning process since they offer learning solutions to learning-disabled students via Apps that may support various disabilities (Ismaili & Ibrahimi, 2016). The positive results obtained in inclusive educational environments indicate the significance role of mobile learning in reference of long-term advancing of technology-based learning solutions.

## 4.2 Theoretical Foundations

Assistive technology can also be planned by a team and this will make schools utilize their resources more effectively to enhance learning among students. Such mobile gadgets as tablets and smartphones are currently gaining popularity as a substitute to conventional assistive technology, particularly in less developed nations. Such devices can as well be used in the form of learning aids by means of special applications that may be provided with the help of such gadgets to students with various impairments. Research also indicated that learning through mobile devices can be effective in inclusive classrooms and this has stimulated further formulation of solutions based on technology in learning.

### 4.2.1 *Universal Design for Learning (UDL)*

The concept of constructivist learning is closely connected with Universal Design of Learning (UDL), because both approaches focus on the variability of learners and the need of flexible type of learning paraments. UDL aims at providing various options in the engagement, representation, and expression so that diverse learners can be supported in modern all-embracing learning settings (Dalton, 2017). The methodology is compatible with the constructivist methods that are based on creating a learner-centered experience in which the constructive knowledge is built through the interactions with the material, the teacher, and the peers (PourhoseinGilakjani et al., 2013). The strategies used in UDL are directed to the creation of expert learners by engaging individuals and motivating them through personal experience being important components of constructivist actions. The paradigm-shifting focus of UDL of taking one-size-fits-all instructions and turning it into differentiated and accommodating learning is close to the constructivist emphasis objective of developing active and individualized learning. With the help of UDL frameworks, educators will be able to make their practices as inclusive as possible, therefore, accommodating the learning needs of disabled learners (Dalton, 2017). Additionally, the empirical evidence indicates that both UDL and constructivist approach will profoundly affect the engagement and self-regulation of the learners. As an example, learning analytics combined with constructivist designs were demonstrated to have positive effects on students, fostering their engagement as well as self-regulation abilities, which is why the combination of both frameworks has synergetic properties (Banihashem et al., 2021). Besides, introducing technology as the positive solution to the problem of designing more inclusive and engaging digital learning environments to UDL fits the constructivist views. It is through such integrations that various learning processes could be attained and efficiency of educational technology could be achieved by rendering appropriate educational theories (PourhoseinGilakjani et al., 2013).

### 4.2.2 *Constructivist Learning Theory*

A well-known approach to education is the Constructivist Learning Theory, which focuses on the active meaning that a learner helps create about him or herself and his or her knowledge. Constructivism also considers that learners develop knowledge basing on all their experiences and interactions with the surrounding world unlike the traditional methods which believe that knowledge is passively delivered to the learner. The notion that learners will act based upon the prior knowledge and experiences in the learning process is central in the constructivist theory. This makes it important to know about the backgrounds of learners and being able to make their education pertinent to their lives. Constructivism has made an impact in many areas, among them being mathematics, science, music, and computer science learning. In mathematics education, an alternative paradigm offered by it, is that students would learn deeper and learn mathematical concepts by solving problem first and thinking critically, instead of memorization. And, again, in science teaching, constructivist-based methods recommend that instead of noticing merely the contents, as has been primarily done, attention should be paid to the methodology of the presentation of concepts in order to achieve a better understanding of scientific concepts (Yager & Lutz, 1994). The practice of the theory also applies to adult learning where it applies to personal sense-making and active investigations of self-directed learning. Constructivism also finds its way in distance and digital education where it assists in the designing of educational technologies that fabricates genuine, dynamic, and interactive complexes of learning. Although widely accepted constructivism has its critic. Others claim that it provides incomplete or distorted perceptions about learning and thus, some constructivist assertions are not different substantially with the existing educational theories. The main operating principles of constructivism recommend the student-centered type of learning and place less emphasis on the teacher giving in much content but encouraging the students to pursue, question and synthesize knowledge actively. The theory still affects how education reforms, instructional tactics, and instructional practices are made in various education settings (Shively, 2015).

### 4.2.3 Experiential and Situated Learning Theories

The experiential and situated learning theories can provide a particular essential role in developing technology-enhanced disability clinical education. An experiential learning that engages the students in a more practical experience is one of the central aspects of clinical education where practice-reflection learning processes are central. The practice of preparing them to situations similar to what can be encountered in the workplace can be particularly useful to students since it teaches them how theoretical concepts can be utilized in the practical spheres thus, it is of particular importance in clinical settings where students will have to interact with patients and disabled people (Kee et al., 2023). Situated learning theory follows this by adding another emphasis to learning in the context in which it will be used. According to this learning approach, the ability to acquire knowledge in a real-life clinical environment is at the core of acquiring professional competence and insight (Patton et al., 2013). Technological integration using assistive machines and online platforms facilitates the experiential learning process and allows students to better expose themselves to the clinical practice, especially those dealing with disabled groups. The integration of the immersive-technology such as augmented and virtual reality in clinical education has the potential to create the real-life setting that the students could experience and make the reflective experience environments with regard to Kolb experiential learning model. Such technologies allow students to take an active part of the process, abstract concepts, and feel the results without facing any of the consequences of clinical mistakes in the real world (Kee et al., 2023). To sum it up, the combination of the theory of experiential learning and of situational learning with contemporary technological devices during the disability clinical education process improves this process. It offers a sound theoretical basis of enhancing the skills required to conduct professional practice in the field of disability services, which equips the learners with effective preparations in fulfilling various needs during clinical practice. Although I would not be able to produce a full essay, the following describes what is learnt about the incorporations of these theories with technology in clinical education given the available literature.

### 4.2.4 Socio-Technical Systems Theory

Technologizing the disability clinical education based on Socio-technical Systems Theory implies comprehending the intricate relationship, in which social and technological elements participate in the educational context. This procedure considers the opportunities as well as the challenges of such integrations. Socio-technical Systems Theory (STST) having very special role in comprehending the interactive nature of the diverse elements of a certain system (i.e., people, technology and organizational structures). The implementation of STST in disability clinical education implies the comprehension of the relationships among technological tools, the educators, disabled students and the structure of the education system itself. The trick is in ensuring that education structures are designed to enable a comprehensive learning experience to the disabled students. Among these is disability competency training, which is about the expertise that healthcare providers have regarding the lives and needs of people with disability. The research notes that although a majority of medical schools say they teach core competencies pertaining to disability, the level and depth of such teaching differ greatly. When implementing the topic of comprehensive disability competency training in medical education, structural changes are necessary, such as modification of the curriculum to include the required competencies in a systematic way. Also, improvements in assistive technologies (AT) provide radical opportunities in terms of better educational and psychological outcomes among disabled students (Mcnicholl et al., 2019, 2020). AT may make students strong by allowing academic participation, facilitating self-efficacy, and well-being. Nevertheless, it is possible to note that AT effectiveness is determined by proper training and support, emphasizing on the socio-technical facet as both technological devices and educational support systems should be regarded as parts of a system aligned as per requirements of the students (Mcnicholl et al., 2019). Moreover, the influence of the socio-technical systems may be discussed in the context of the hybrid socio-technical system framework which unites various knowledge bases and creates constructive tension. The systems pose particular opportunities and challenges in establishing sustainable transformation in the conditions of education, where inclusivity and diversity are essential (Balanzó-Guzman & Ramos-Mejía, 2023). On the whole, the implementation of STST in disability clinical education is associated not only with the involvement of technological advances such as AI and AT but with a thorough awareness of the social dynamics of a given field. This involves the training of the educators, policymakers and the supporting staffs in how to accommodate a student with disability in effective ways. Integrative education has the potential to make education more democratic and minimize the difference between the kids so that there can be an inclusive and needs-based learning culture (Bulathwela et al., 2024).

## 4.3 Technological Innovations in Clinical Education

Clinical education has undergone substantial changes due to technological innovation and learning by several hundred percent as it has brought changes in a variety of innovative devices and approaches to learning experiences and clinical procedures. The utilization of simulation-based training (SBT) is one of the most evident instances, and it has been adopted as one of the pillars of medical education. SBT uses high fidelity manikins; the use of virtual reality, under patient scenarios, and hybrid simulations creates a secure and controlled learning space, fostering the development of both clinical and soft skills. Such an approach leads to an increase in skills, minimizes errors, and allows performing the same workplaces again without posing any danger to real patients, with a positive impact on patient security and clinical results in the end (Elendu et al., 2024). Microscope technologies such as virtual and optical microscopes have also been instrumental especially in the case of teaching and learning of histology and pathology. More popular especially among medical students when compared to optical microscopes, virtual microscopes (ability to view digital slides by use of whole slide imaging, WSI) have become popular learning modalities. This technology allows online viewing and other interactive capabilities like pan-and-zoom to increase the learning, like the traditional slide examination, but without being limited by it. In the topic of regional anesthesia education, modern teaching now encompasses web-based education and simulation-based teaching and alternate reality systems. These technologies are of use in competency-based progression and offer new methods to educate and evaluate medical trainees efficiently and with a high quality of education which can be adjusted to the new developments of medical knowledge and practice (Ramlogan et al., 2021). Another emerging technology that has positive perception among the postgraduate trainees is artificial intelligence (AI). It is hoped that AI would improve research and quality improvement competencies as well as decrease clinical workload. Nevertheless, medical curricula express a need to have rigorous AI training to make the most use of it in clinical learning without spoiling the fate of practicing critical skills (instructive assessment and practical skills) development (Banerjee et al., 2021). In addition to this, to tackle the problem of offering real patients as a learning experience, livestreaming of clinical experiences has also been introduced and especially amidst the COVID-19 pandemic. Livestreamed experiences increase access to clinical placements, standardizes learning experience and in general student's take it well. However, issues like maintaining engagement in learners and addressing such technical problems as connectivity still persist (Gomez et al., 2024). An example of systemic innovation in medical education is Accelerating Change in Medical Education (ACE) initiative to medical education proposed by the American Medical Association, focusing on approaches to competency-based education, pathway and place technology capability, and the enrichment of learning environments. This type of undertaking plays a critical role in spreading education-based innovations and enhancing medical training on a wide level.

### 4.3.1 Assistive Technologies

A big role in creating more inclusive and accessible medical education lies in assistive technologies. Screen readers allow blind students to read online material and voice-to-text programs make it easier to take notes in case of students who lack mobility. Adaptive keyboards accommodate students with diverse physical requirements so that they are able to perform well as they communicate with online learning contents. Simulation on wheel chairs grants everyone an opportunity to have hands-on training, and haptic feedback devices add advantage to the learning process to the students with sensory defects. These technologies in sum will make an equal learning environment in medical study. The use of simulations in the practice revolutionized clinical education and learning since it offers a structured and secured environment where students perform, can practice, and execute their clinical abilities (Elendu et al., 2024). Virtual patients and high fidelity manikins present their opportunities to have realistic situations and train the students, and augmented and virtual reality technologies provide the learners with immersion in realistic clinical scenarios. It is a scenario-based interactive simulation that permits students to make choices and see results on a risk-free environment. Many avenues of knowledge about medicine are now open in the form of e-learning and mobile learning platforms, and remote learning and collaboration have become possible with MOOCs and learning management systems. Tele-education and synchronous learning possibilities allow communicating in real time between the instructors and enrollees, no matter the geographical boundaries. The adoption of the concept of artificial intelligence in clinical training has played a very positive role in the learning process, including a number of key innovations:

i. Feedback systems with the help of AI: These offer personalized feedback to students in clinical simulations or learning practice in real time to inform students about the areas they need to work and strengthen the proper methods.
ii. Revision and clarification chatbots: AI-based chatbots also provide round-the-clock support and support students with answers, explanations, and revision of tricky medical concepts.
iii. Personalized learning pathways: AI algorithms can examine the record of student performance to provide personalized learning plans, working on weak points and respond to unique student learning styles.

iv. Adaptive-learning technologies: The way through reshape the content and challenge of learning materials according to the performance of the students and guarantee them pleasant challenge and involvement.
v. Natural language processing of medical documentation: AI can be used to teach students about proper medical documentation through analysis of the mistakes of student-written medical reports and case studies as well as adjusting these students on their writing technique.
vi. Virtual patient interactions: These virtual patients are AI-driven, which enables them to recreate realistic clinical situations with students having access to a safe situation to diagnose and plan treatment.
vii. Performance tracking and analytics: AI-based programs track the performance of the students over time, highlight the trends and give feedback to both the learners and educators to further improve on their respective performances.
viii. Intelligent tutoring systems: These are AI platforms that use Artificial Intelligence to offer individual attention, as well as assistance to learners, based on their mentality dispositions and rate of learning.
ix. Automated grading and assessment: AI make the assessment and grading of students incredibly simple and thus fast as the AI grades the student based on the performance in the simulations and written examinations.
x. Skill decay prediction: The AI can predict when the skills of a learner are likely to start becoming rusty and specific course refreshers can be provided to ensure that the skill is retained.

## 4.4 Enhancing Accessibility Through Technology

Inclusion and learning of disabled students with the help of assistant technologies is the main idea of technological increase in accessibility of disability clinical education. The use of assistive technologies (AT) shows (Fig. 4.2) its valuable contribution in the field of higher education, providing an educational experience, promoting academic self-efficacy, and influencing psychosocial parameters, Enhancing learners' self-efficacy, adaptability, and emotional well-being (Mcnicholl et al., 2020). This is necessary as disabled students struggle to get appropriate education to their needs.

Furthermore, the development of mobile learning environments as an alternative to conventional assistive technologies can resolve the problem of availability and cost in those areas where they have minimal access to special equipment. Open-source mobile applications are also a solution that can enhance the education of persons with various types of disabilities and provide both students and an otherwise costly option (Ismaili & Ibrahimi, 2016). Technology is also very significant in improving physical accessibility in learning contexts in addition to the direct education support it offers. Accessibility mobile applications allow individuals with disabilities to find their way around buildings and facilities in support of independence and inclusion (Apostolidou & Fokaides, 2023). Developing the unified platform of the app assessment makes them more reliable and accessible, which encourages inclusivity. As

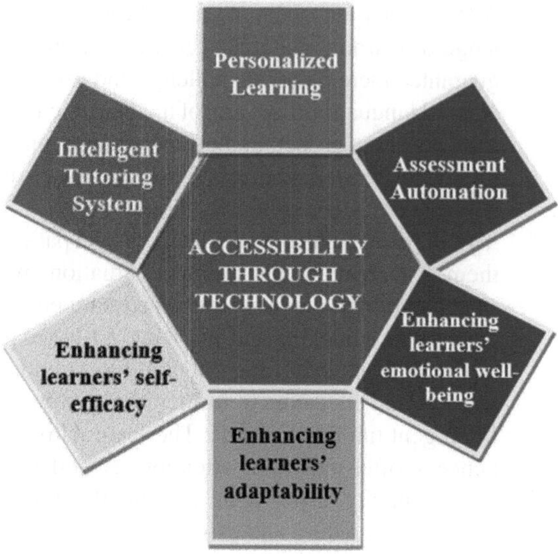


**Fig. 4.2** Enhancing accessibility through technology

well, the use of the Universal Design for Learning (UDL) framework can maximize the functionality of assistive technology in secondary education establishments. UDL encourages the personalization of the educational resources to suit different educational requirements, which coupled with the use of the assistive technology can improve educational achievements of the disabled students. But the limited staff training, negative attitude, lack of proper assessment and funding have been an obstacle in assistive technology implementation and there is need to coordinate efforts to address the obstacles (Copley & Ziviani, 2004). Making improvements in policy and professional development would help address these barriers in reference to make the educational experiences of younger persons with disabilities optimum. In essence, technology is transformational to the inclusion of disabled students into clinical environments within the present education system.

### *4.4.1 Digital Accessibility Standards (WCAG 2.1)*

The Web-Content Accessibility-Guidelines (WCAG) 2.1 are very important as managed by the Web-Accessibility-Initiative (WAI) that decides at developing guidelines to develop at web content available to everyone, including disabled persons. These guidelines are introductory to the fore going designs which integrate accessibility as an important component of web platform design and development. WCAG 2.1 concepts revolve around four broad POUR (perceivable, operable, understandable and robust) principles. These guidelines enable web developers to carry out web design and develop content that is easy to read, listen to, and utilize by any individual possible (Ara & Sik-Lanyi, 2022; Iniesto & Rodrigo, 2024). However, the recent studies emphasize the necessity to guarantee web accessibility in many areas, including health care and education. To illustrate this, the availability of a government websites that were hosting essential health information was critical in the COVID-19 pandemic. It was found that there were significant differences in the likelihood of meeting the WCAG 2.0, 2.1, demonstrating that most websites were not entirely accessible, which would make accessibility difficult to people with disabilities (Ara & Sik-Lanyi, 2022). The study of web accessibility has demonstrated that there are certain problems that are repeated on various platforms. Among them, one can point out issues in the structure of the websites, the lack of relevance of the information presented, insufficient design elements (color contrast, font size, and so on) that all fall within the WCAG (Ara & Sik-Lanyi, 2022). Moreover, research results demonstrated that automated tools, although helpful, tend to find or misclassify WCAG compliance problems and justifying the multifaceted nature of comprehending WCAG standards adequately (Iniesto & Rodrigo, 2024). As a reaction to these concerns, calls have been issued upon the empirical corroboration of the accessibility norms. Some have reasoned that WCAG guidelines must be integrated with the actual usability testing and include a wider representation of accessibility. It would not only guarantee the technical requirements of websites, but also the functional usability various people are likely to have. With the change of digital landscapes, constant improvement of the issues of accessibility is required, and it is necessary to create all the platforms accessible and equal to everyone. The certification of WCAG 2.1 has shown its effectiveness in integrating the item in areas such as the Accessible Platform for Respiratory Therapies (PAR) that affirms accessibility in the medical arena executed through the telemedical concept and user-focused design.

### *4.4.2 The Text-To-Speech and Speech Recognition Tools*

Machine learning & deep learning technology has improved the text-to-speech (TTS) and speech recognition technology greatly. Text-to-Speech (TTS) Technologies: The technology of TTS is concentrated on transferring written wording to the speech. Deep learning has made TTS systems much better as speech is near-human and of high quality. These systems tend to use a large number of text-speech pairs to evolve feature representations that may serve the purpose of bridging both text and speech. The modern TTS models aim not only at high-quality synthesis but also focus on expressive output, which can convey various emotions and talking styles, similar to the speech of people (Barakat et al., 2024). TTS systems have shifted direction toward being multilingual, multispeaker, and now address problems in resource-low languages using models such as ZMM-TTS, which employ self-supervised learning (Gong et al., 2024). Speech recognition tools: When this tool uses Automatic Speech Recognition (ASR) technology, it will translate what is spoken aloud into text. It is an emerging field, which is already applied in solving communication barriers associated with different languages, and as well improving smart devices interactions (Vashisht et al., 2021). The older ASR systems were based on complex algorithms such as hidden Markov model (HMM) but have evolved to deep learning framework. The modern systems use the concept of neural networks to cope with the intricacy of the human speaking behavior more effectively. To enhance recognition and gain sufficient accuracy levels, especially when recognizing dysarthric speech, more simultaneous modalities are incorporated into advanced models, including audio-visual fusion (Qian et al., 2023). Innovative approaches such as deep fusion involving the incorporation of outside language models have been promising in making ASR systems more accurate and applicable in low-resource languages. The two technologies have further advanced and in the latest inventions, the technologies base some of their trials on deep reinforcement learning, zero-shot learning and using the new discoveries in the design of neural networks to expand their applications to more linguistic setups and enhance performance in linguistic setups that these two technologies operate as well.

### *4.4.3 Audible Descriptions and Captioning Service*

Captioning services and audio description are important in providing multimedia content to handicapped people, with deafness, hard of hearing, or visual impairment. Captioning is the printing of words on a screen or a video that describes what people speak and can be used by people with impaired hearing ability and audio description has a descriptive voice describing relevant visual images and can be used by people who cannot see well.

i. Advances in Audio Captioning: The past decade has witnessed that the development of considerable concern in automated audio captioning, on the back of advances in deep learning. It is the process of creating textual accounts to the audio snippets with the help of a custom neural network structure and training approaches.
ii. Universal Design Challenges: In fact, existent practices in closed captioning and audio description do not comply with universal design. This is more so because they are incorporated late in the production process and this may result to absence of control and creative input by the directors. This means that in order to improve the efficacy and artistic design of such services, it should be involved in the initial stages of the content development.
iii. Video Captioning Strategies: In case of videos, the dynamic and syntax-directional hierarchy-based attention networks are going to be developed. These methods have also sought to enhance captioning placement as well as accuracy based on visual cues as well as organizing sentence structure context by offering superior assistance to the hearing impaired.
iv. Audio Description for the Visually Impaired: Active systems such as CineAD attempt to automate the process of audio description of video materials therewith relying on available scripts and closed-captions, which could counteract the high rates and time-related requirements, which are often a reality when manually

creating audio description (Campos et al., 2018). Moreover, lightweight video captioning models are under development to help visually impaired people in describing audio of the surrounding in real time on implemented platforms (Yousif & Al-Jammas, 2024).

v. Newer Technologies and Benchmarking: As an example, the creation of tasks like text-audio and audio-text retrieval benchmarks holds some potential to develop the field. Such a cross-modal method gives an opportunity to retrieve audio content which corresponds to textual descriptions and vice versa, an essential feature to provide more intuitive and more accessible audio description services (Koepke et al., 2023).

### *4.4.4 Available Electronic Health Records (EHRs)*

Available EHRs has many benefits in the promotion of patient participation and better health care. Healthcare systems enable patients to view their electronic health record, which leads to patient empowerment, enhances patient safety and patient care satisfaction. Easy access of records by the patient will enhance interaction between the patient and medical officers and the patient will become actively involved in his or her health choices and care plans. Also, the availability of EHRs facilitates the administrative process, minimizes medical errors, and enhances the coordination of care as these tools help to make healthcare providers knowledgeable of detailed information about patients. Reception and adoption of accessible EHRs are however not without difficulties. The issue of privacy and security is one of the matters of concern, and the sensitive character of health data requires the high level of protection against uncontrolled access and cyberattacks. Maintaining a careful balance between sharing data and protecting patient privacy is vital, as patients are less likely to trust healthcare systems that fail to safeguard their personal information. Domestic budgets and differing levels of willingness by healthcare providers to make records available are the other obstacles to the implementation of it widely. Another issue would be interoperability as in the case of EHR systems, data exchange between various healthcare centers and systems is usually hampered by the absence of common sets of protocols. This negatively affects the seamless integration required in care of the comprehensive patient care (Rathert et al., 2019). Promising ventures to overcome these challenges are the embrace of blockchain technology that would provide a secure decentralized model to EHR systems to increase data security and interoperability (Benaich et al., 2023). Training is also needed to enable medical workers and patients to understand how to move in and use an EHR system. By guaranteeing that patients are capable of comprehending their health records, an improved health outcome and a more significant decision-making can be achieved.

## 4.5 Case Studies and Best Practices

Application of digital tools in clinical instruction of disabilities can help with the learning processes and yield better results to the students and patients. The Inclusive Simulation Initiative at Harvard Medical School, University of Sydney Disability-Inclusive Clinical Education Program, and the University of Open University UK Virtual Clinics Educational Programs of Hearing-Impaired are all the examples of the new solutions to the inclusive learning in the context of technology and delivery techniques. Also, the implementation of Augmented Reality (AR) in physiotherapy study at the University of Toronto can be considered as one of the examples of the application of an advanced technological means to promote educational experience. The Inclusive Simulation Initiative of Harvard Medical School is aimed at developing simulation-based learning that is permeable to a wide range of learner backgrounds, abilities and views. This measure will increase the clinical expertise, organizations in cultural competence in students through the application of lifelike simulation to capture a wide scope of patients with different physical and mental capabilities. With the help of such an initiative, the inclusive simulation becomes part of the curriculum and prepares medical students to offer effective and compassionate care to all patient groups. The Disability-Inclusive Clinical Education Program at the University of Sydney is aimed at getting the clinical education approach both accessible to and accommodating disabled students. Such a program combines specific student support services, customized learning methods and adaptive technologies to support clinical student training environments with varied needs. This program will enable disabled students as well as enhance the learning capacity of the other students through a culture of diversity and acceptance. The application of AR in the University of Toronto physiotherapy training process is an indication of the opportunities of technology to transform health education. AR apps have compensated this lack of interactivity and immersion as the lessons offered are interactive and immersive where students gain the opportunity to visualize and interact with anatomical structures and treatment methods in a virtual setting. AR-based methodologies have been demonstrated useful in the education of such complex topics as training in anatomy and clinical decision-making, and may be used to supplement conventional learning approaches to help increase learning and memorization (Lucena-Anton et al., 2022). Finally, the Open University UK has adopted Virtual Clinics Hearing Impaired Students showing how a distance learning care program in medical education can be inclusive of students with impairments. In virtual clinics, the hearing impaired students get the chance to experience clinics as they would in the real world, only that there is no such possibility of such students using the traditional strategies of communicating through hearing and sound. The strategy will fit within the general trends in the field of virtual care, which have demonstrated potential in expanding access and decreasing the barriers to leading to specialized learning and care.

## 4.6 Impact on Learning Outcomes

The influences of different educational issues on the learning performances are many-sided and interconnected. Student engagement and motivation, skill retention, performance, self-efficacy, confidence in clinical environments, peer collaboration and interprofessional learning are just a few of the essential factors as given in Table 4.1.

### *4.6.1 Student Engagement and Motivation*

Student engagement in the educational environment is very instrumental in academic learning and achievement. Gamification is revealed to stimulate great motivation

**Table 4.1** Educational strategies that shape student learning outcomes

| Factor | Description | Impact on learning outcomes | Supporting references |
|---|---|---|---|
| Student engagement and motivation | Involves students' active participation and emotional investment in learning; gamification and online activities enhance it | Increases academic performance, interest, and motivation in learning | Fuentes-Riffo et al., (2023) and Wang et al., (2023) |
| Skill retention and performance | Influenced by self-regulated learning strategies (SRLS) and the integration of technology in learning | Improves knowledge retention and practical performance through active and autonomous learning | Anthonysamy et al., (2020) and Memon et al., (2022) |
| Self-efficacy and confidence | Refers to students' belief in their own capabilities to succeed, especially in clinical environments | Predicts academic performance and confidence in practical/clinical tasks | Saks (2024) |
| Peer collaboration & interprofessional learning | Involves teamwork and shared learning experiences across disciplines | Enhances broader understanding, teamwork skills, and academic success through cooperative efforts | Saks (2024) |
| Integrated educational practices | Combines gamification, SRLS, technology, and collaboration in a supportive learning environment | Leads to holistic academic and personal growth by fostering engagement, motivation, and performance | Anthonysamy et al., (2020) and Saks (2024) |

among students and make them more engaged, so academic performance could be improved (Fuentes-Riffo et al., 2023). Owing to implementation of gaming aspects within the learning settings, Game-like experiences can make learning more engaging and motivating for students, interest, & eventually, the learning results. In addition, online learning activity can be used as a positive predictor of academic achievement, especially in the case of its interaction with strategies such as inquiry and reflective learning (Wang et al., 2023).

### 4.6.2 Skill Retention and Performance

Skill retention and general performance depend on a matter of factors, such as self-regulated-learning-strategies (SRLS) and the use of technology. SRLS play critical roles in assisting students in regulating their learning processes effectively, hence improving academic and functional performance too (Anthonysamy et al., 2020). Also, technology through interactive and self-regulated learning presents an intermediate influence on the performance of the students implying the relevance of technology in enhancing student achievement (Memon et al., 2022).

### 4.6.3 Self-Efficacy and Confidence in Clinical Settings:

Self-efficacy, which is a belief that a person has in his or her capacity to accomplish something in a given circumstance, is critical in terms of goals achievement and determination of grades. It makes a predictive influence on the expected grades and learning outcomes based on the motivational aspects of online learning conditions (Saks, 2024). The self-belief is vital in the clinical environment where confidence could directly affect the performance and patient care.

### 4.6.4 Peer Collaboration and Interprofessional Learning

Adoption of cooperative learning among peers within different disciplines (interprofessional learning) improves the learning outcomes, as the practice enables the learners to acquire a broader view and learn to work as a team. Though particular researches concerning interprofessional learning were not described in the given environment, approaches aimed at enhancing learner engagement such as the use of different types of collaboration is a dominant way of approaching success in educational processes. The combined impact of motivational, engagement and learning strategies in academic achievements is closely reflected in these studies. To improve the retention of skills and the performance of the students, effective educational practice must include such elements as gamification, self-regulation of learning, and use of technology. The combination of all these methods can provide support and inspiring atmosphere in education, which is a key to both academic and personal growth (Anthonysamy et al., 2020; Saks, 2024).

## 4.7 Barriers to Integration

Implementation of new systems and technologies in academic institutions in diverse settings is normally hampered by a number of challenges. A crucial obstacle to this is technological infrastructure and cost. These may include absence of standardization, high costs of IT resources, and infrastructure issues which are especially problematic in the low-resource settings and developing countries (Harris et al., 2021). The lack of adequate support on the institutional level and limited financial resources contributes to the unwillingness to implement novel tools, such as online learning platforms or AI technologies, and forms a massive obstacle in the general integration process. Another major challenge is faculty preparedness and training shortage. Although faculty members in universities may appreciate that technological tools have the potential of improving learning and research, they are unable to use them effectively owing to the fact that they are not familiar with the tools and lack in knowledge about using the tools because they have not been trained. It is important to overcome these challenges with training programs attuned to the needs of the faculty and boosting their flexibility (Valle-Flórez et al., 2021). In addition, all institutions are very different in terms of preparedness, where the willingness to implement such technologies prevails in some institutions, and organizational and cultural resistance becomes the barriers in others (Adams et al., 2023). Cultural barrier to change is the reluctance to adopt new things and it can cause integration to take very long. The basis of resistance is the fear of ownership of outputs and changes in operations which can interfere with the current norms and cultures at the institution. This is further augmented by a rather skeptical attitude towards the overall use of the emerging technologies such as the telemedicine or the AI models in at least some educational environments which can also be burdened by an issue linked with possible privacy and ethical concerns as yet (Batsis et al., 2020). Lastly, the policy and accreditation limitations have become very instrumental either in supporting or preventing integration. The necessity to comply with the existing policies and accreditation bodies also implies that academic institutions usually have to face regulatory issues. This is further aggravated in jurisdictions where the law is yet to fully capture the new technologies being incorporated thereby restraining the extent of its potential use. Meanwhile, there are ways to address these impediments, such as building collaboration, creating detailed guidelines, and providing specific training courses; however, due to its complexity, the integration work will have to involve finer strategies based on the needs and limitations of specific institutions (Adams et al., 2023).

## 4.8 Ethical and Legal Considerations

Digital simulation Ethical and legal issues There is a wide scope of aspects related to digital simulation in terms of appropriateness and legality such as information privacy and security, anti-discrimination and equity, informed consent, and accommodations, as opposed to modifications. As far as data privacy and security are concerned, it is necessary to provide confidentiality and integrity of sensitive data, especially in such settings as telemedicine and mental health programs (Gooding & Kariotis, 2021). As an example, the General-Data-Protection-Regulation (GDPR) in the European Union offers a framework on how to protect personal data and ensures that the entities setting the protection need to employ effective data protection strategies. This regulation emphasizes the aspect of obeying to safeguard user data on digital simulations. An important consideration is equity and non-discrimination especially in research technologies and mental health care. The ethical approach to research requires that it is not biased on grounds of a particular group of people and it must represent an equal opportunity and representation of diverse model in digital simulations and information-driven technologies (Tzafestas, 2018). Algorithmic accountability can be critical toward avoiding biases that might give rise to discriminatory results. The subject of informed consent is of great ethical concern particularly in the digital environments and simulations. It entails making the study participants aware of what the study is all about, and allowing the individuals to participate out of their will. The concern to guarantee the participants that understand how their information will be used and their rights in the digital domain is even more significant in digital simulations (Yellowlees et al., 2012). Accommodations versus modifications debate revolves around the notion of adapting or transforming digitalized simulations to fulfill the variances of the users. Accommodations are the alterations or the improvement of the current setting in order to facilitate the participation, but not to change a nature of the activity, whereas the alteration of the activity or the material it is called the modification. One should balance out so that the integrity of the simulation is respected but everyone should feel accessible and included (Clark et al., 2018).

## 4.9 Policy and Institutional Frameworks

Technology incorporation in disability clinical education entails numerous policy and institutional models that aim at creating the culture of inclusive and equitable educational settings. The most important findings and models can be taken out of the recent literature in this sphere as in Table 4.2:

i. **Disability Models from Diagnosis to Social Inclusion**: The great stress is laid on the move-away from a medico-model of disability based on deficits to a social model that lays stress on ability and access. Literature based on social models promote fulfilling changes in such education systems and emphasize the significance of inclusive educational practices.

ii. **Special Education Policy Inclusive Education Legislation**: Ideas like as the personal with Disabilities-Education-Act (IDEA) and others provide that the most comprehensive provision of educational services possible should be provided in inclusive classrooms. The application of inclusive practice models of service provision, like those followed by the speech-language-pathologists, contributes to the creation of the educationally relevant individualized education plans (IEPs) that fit the schooling services to the requirements of the students within the general learning setting (Heilmann et al., 2023).
iii. **Assistive-Technology Integration**: Human-Activity-Assistive-Technology model underlines the importance of assistive technologies in helping individuals with disabilities participate fully in education. This model combines the occupational therapy social concepts and increases the utility of assistive technologies in clinical settings (Giesbrecht, 2013). When incorporated into national disability plans and education interventions, assistive technologies can reduce the disparities in infrastructural and access-related gaps within the educational environment, as it was observed in the study on visual impairments (Kisanga & Kisanga, 2020).
iv. **Challenges and Barriers**: Although policies have been presented that provoke inclusivism, physical, cultural, and institutional barriers that restrict the transition to inclusive education prevail. These obstacles point to instances of mismatches between the meaning of policies (as mentioned in the European Disability Strategy) and these policies and practices, which require further improvement of inclusive educational practice and policies.
v. **Institutional Readiness and Faculty Involvement**: The institutional structures should also counter faculty preparedness and availability to apply the inclusive education initiatives. Investigations indicate that not all faculty members are ready to teach inclusively and require professional work on educational strategies and a change of awareness about new legislative reality (Lopatina et al., 2023).

### *4.9.1 Guidelines on Assistive Technology Issued by WHO*

The World Health Organization (WHO) has come up with GATE (Global-Cooperation on Assistive Technology) program aimed at ensuring greater accessibility to rich-quality and affordable-assistive-technology (AT) to those with different disabilities, diseases, and age-related health conditions. GATE program is an attempt to target the needs of millions of people that need the assistive devices in their everyday life (Boot et al., 2017). The compilation of a list of assistive products is one of the most important elements of the GATE program because it establishes priorities in the provision of products on the basis of the most urgent need at the population level. This is essential as the problem of many people with intellectual-disabilities being ignored in this sphere has been in existence where there is a need to pay more

**Table 4.2** Policy and institutional framework

| Key area | Description | Impact on disability clinical education |
|---|---|---|
| Disability models: from diagnosis to social inclusion | Transition from a deficit-based medical model to a social model focusing on ability and accessibility | Promotes inclusive educational practices and emphasizes student potential and rights |
| Special & inclusive education policies | Laws like IDEA mandate inclusive education and individualized support through IEPs tailored to student needs in general education settings | Facilitates structured support for students with disabilities in mainstream classrooms |
| Assistive technology integration | The Human-Activity-Assistive-Technology (HAAT) model integrates assistive tools to enhance participation in education | Reduces access disparities; supports equal learning opportunities for students with disabilities |
| Challenges and barriers | Despite policies, many barriers (physical, cultural, institutional) hinder full inclusion due to policy-practice gaps | Highlights the need for consistent policy application and continued policy development |
| Institutional readiness & faculty involvement | Institutions must ensure faculty are trained, aware, and prepared for inclusive teaching | Lack of readiness among faculty signals the need for professional development and awareness programs |

attention to such groups under the GATE concept (Boot et al., 2017). Besides, the initiative by WHO is in line with the global systems targeting the availability of assistive technologies and making them affordable. Proposals have been given to come up with an international standard of the AT provision to improve the accessibility and quality of these technologies all over the world. The stated standards are also expected to direct policy formulation, systems, and even service delivery processes to enhance access to AT (De Witte et al., 2018). Much as this is being done accessibility to assistive technology in the developing world is quite painful. Obstacles like unavailability of relevant services and poor policies are major. CRPD gives the duties of governments to fulfill the AT needs of its people, but in non-developed countries find it difficult to implement the Convention. Thus, the research and activities connected with the rule policies, service-based delivery and cooperation from all over world are required in order to address these needs efficiently.

## 4.10 UN CRPD and Right to Education

United Nations Convention on the Rights of Persons with Disabilities (CRPD) has an essential role in providing the international benchmark of rights of the persons with disabilities, especially educational rights, found under Article 24. It highlights the value of inclusive learning environments and insists that embracing inclusion should not come at the cost of adequate support for children with significant disabilities (Byrne, 2019). The CRPD invents a system through which states can guarantee rights of people based on disability and it also aims at redefining the rights in a social disability model so that it does not remain a formality as is the case in the general human rights conventions. When speaking of national plans, such countries as India, the USA and the UK have already started to comply with the contents of the CRPD, though each of these presents its difficulties. An example is the case of India which ratified the CRPD in the year 2007 and as a consequence, enacted the Rights of Persons with Disabilities (RPwD) Act in 2016. The RPwD act represented a movement to a more inclusive policy of a biopsychosocial model of disability with its setbacks in disability recognition, including challenges related to mental well-being and the ability to make informed legal choices. Additionally, the effect of CRPD in the amendment and reform of mental health laws has also been felt in a number of countries with the change in mental capacity law, treatment without consent and civil detention. These notwithstanding, each jurisdiction has a different practical implementation, and there are claims over how meaningful inclusive education is in relation to the mandates of the CRPD (De Beco, 2016). It is also evident that a significant emphasis has been placed on the necessity of constant efforts and the governmental intervention to mainstream the disability rights and achieve the realistic social change, which involves the development of instruments and strategies to move toward the inclusive education (De Beco, 2016). Moreover, CRPD-related legislation provides a possibility of gradual changes in mental health law and draws focus to the necessity of the systems that not only ensure legal competence but the comprehensive engagement of people with disabilities in the life of society (Kelly, 2016). CRPD has had an essential impact on education and disability rights policy all over the world as it promotes states to reconsider their policies and practices in more inclusive directions. Nevertheless, there are still some issues with properly applying such principles, especially when it comes to education systems and mental health law reforms (Byrne, 2019).

## 4.11 Future Directions and Global Networks for Inclusive Clinical Education

Developments of machine learning (ML) and AI in adaptive learning systems, blockchain as a credentialing system and portfolio, proliferation of XR-based clinical laboratories, and the creation of international systems of inclusive clinical education all show much potential in having a positive impact on both the educational and clinical training settings.

i. ***AI and Machine Learning in Adaptive Learning Systems***: Applying intelligent technologies to personalize and enhance education is not alien and has been heavily used towards developing adaptive learning systems. The technologies allow analyzing data about students to predict performance and raise student engagement and motivation by offering individual learning materials (Akavova et al., 2023). When learning methods are powered by AI, it is common to find algorithms adopting the changing learning style of the student, hence maximizing learning (Essa et al., 2023). Not only does the introduction of AI allow students to enhance their learning experience, but it also gives a helping hand to teachers, who no longer have to resort to manual work regarding administrative processes and can instead receive instant feedback (Sajja et al., 2024).

ii. ***Blockchain to Credentialing and Portfolios***: The blockchain technology is revolutionary in providing educational credentialing in a secure, decentralized, tamper-, peer-, and censorship-free way. It could simplify the verification exercise and make the educational qualifications more visible and transparent (Samala et al., 2024). The self-sovereign identity feature of blockchain specifically helps to design digital credentialing, ensure identity integrity, and ascribe transnational trust to educational credentials (Grech et al., 2021).

iii. ***Growth of XR-powered Clinical Labs***: Extended Reality (XR) such as Virtual-Reality (VR) and Augmented Reality (AR) is emerging in medical education because of the immersive and interactive nature of this growing technology. XR technologies have a great benefit in training settings: they can increase medical procedures realism and create safe practice settings (Morimoto et al., 2022). Such technologies enable simulating surgical procedures and complex clinical situations, which helps to minimize risks and expenses that are involved in clinical training (Arensmeyer et al., 2023).

iv. ***Global Networks of Inclusive Clinical Education***: Globalization has prepared the path to more connected educational networks and this has created an environment that encourages working across borders and sharing knowledge. The establishment of strong international networks could be used to foster inclusive clinical educational by using online platforms of faculties and learners in all over world (Shields, 2013). Such international dynamics will allow exchanging resources, practices, and best training approaches, thus creating a more homogeneous and accessible visual field of healthcare education. In general, the future of both technologies in education and clinical practice will be bright as it will increase personal experiences, security, interaction, and connectivity on a global scale. They also will deal with ethical and technical issues in order to achieve their maximum potential to change methodologies of education and training.

## 4.12 Conclusion & Future Scope

Employing technology in the clinical teaching field of disability can be of many benefits and additionally challenges. Among the most notable ones is the enhancement of inclusion and accessibility that most disabled students would find. Intelligent assistive technologies, including AIoT items, advance everyday life and learning by offering knowledge and helping to make choices (De Freitas et al., 2022). They work with several impairments and have extensive interest in visual impairments and typically via portable devices, wearables, and smartphones with machine-learning models. Nevertheless, there are certain difficulties with the process of integration. The significant obstacle is the absence of an appropriate staff training and assistance in functioning with assistive technologies in educational field. Also, negative attitude of some of the staff members, deficient assessment and planning procedures as well as lack of funds and procedures of acquiring and managing equipment continue to compound the integration (Copley & Ziviani, 2004). The difference in professional development and acquaintance with the opportunities of the existing assistive technologies creates significant limitations in using such technologies and their usefulness. Despite legal provisions under IDEA supporting access to assistive technology, its use in classrooms remains limited—mainly because many educators haven't been properly trained to implement it in meaningful ways (Judge & Simms, 2009). The coverage of AT coursework required by the undergraduate special education teacher licensure programs is roughly one-third, which shows that more encompassing training programs are necessary (Judge & Simms, 2009). When it comes to higher education, despite the fact that disabled students become aware of and use available assistive technologies, the growing need is to make them more inclusive and accessible (Papadopoulos et al., 2024). To progress with equity in care and care delivery in terms of clinical education, the application of the assistive technology should take into consideration the graphical aspects, including inclusive design and investing in infrastructure. Assistive technology is not used in educational settings to its potential, revealing an essential barrier between policy and practice. The difference does not only impact disabled students, but it also has an implication on the level of education and health service delivery. In order to solve this problem, it is utmost necessary to develop the most thorough training systems that would empower teachers with the skill they need to introduce assistive technologies to the setting of varying learning experiences. Moreover, the need to increase the use of more helpful and inclusive assistive technologies in tertiary colleges demonstrates that the issue of user design is significant. Listening to and understanding students with disabilities enables the creation of technology that not only meets their needs but also fosters greater independence and inclusion. Such orientation toward inclusivity and accessibility can eventually translate into better educational results and a higher degree of equality in an educational and healthcare environment.

## References

Adams, D., Azzis, M. S. A., Chuah, K.-M., & Devadason, E. (2023). From novice to navigator: Students' academic help-seeking behaviour, readiness, and perceived usefulness of ChatGPT in learning. *Education and Information Technologies, 29*(11), 13617–13634. https://doi.org/10.1007/s10639-023-12427-8

Akavova, A., Lorsanova, Z., & Temirkhanova, Z. (2023). Adaptive learning and artificial intelligence in the educational space. *E3S Web of Conferences, 451*, 06011. https://doi.org/10.1051/e3sconf/202345106011

Anthonysamy, L., Hew, S.-H., & Koo, A.-C. (2020). Self-regulated learning strategies and non-academic outcomes in higher education blended learning environments: A one decade review. *Education and Information Technologies, 25*(5), 3677–3704. https://doi.org/10.1007/s10639-020-10134-2

Apostolidou, E., & Fokaides, P. A. (2023). Enhancing accessibility: A comprehensive study of current apps for enabling accessibility of disabled individuals in buildings. *Buildings, 13*(8), 2085. https://doi.org/10.3390/buildings13082085

Ara, J., & Sik-Lanyi, C. (2022). Investigation of COVID-19 vaccine information websites across Europe and Asia using automated accessibility protocols. *International Journal of Environmental Research and Public Health, 19*(5), 2867. https://doi.org/10.3390/ijerph19052867

Arensmeyer, J., Feodorovici, P., Schmidt, J., & Schnorr, P. (2023). Extended Reality (XR)—Applications in thoracic surgery. *ZentralblattFürChirurgie - ZeitschriftFür Allgemeine, Viszeral-, Thorax- und Gefäßchirurgie, 148*(4), 367–375. https://doi.org/10.1055/a-2121-6478

Balanzó-Guzmán, A., & Ramos-Mejía, M. (2023). Towards epistemic diversity in sustainability transitions: An exploration of hybrid socio-technical systems. *Sustainability Science, 18*(6), 2511–2531. https://doi.org/10.1007/s11625-023-01370-9

Banerjee, M., Zaman, S., Johns, I., Ross, J., Szram, J., Chappell, D., Chiew, D., Francis, D. P., Linton, N., Patel, K. T., & Cole, G. D. (2021). The impact of artificial intelligence on clinical education: perceptions of postgraduate trainee doctors in London (UK) and recommendations for trainers. *BMC Medical Education, 21*(1). https://doi.org/10.1186/s12909-021-02870-x

Banihashem, S. K., Farrokhnia, M., Badali, M., &Noroozi, O. (2021). The impacts of constructivist learning design and learning analytics on students' engagement and self-regulation. *Innovations in Education and Teaching International* (ahead-of-print), 442–452. https://doi.org/10.1080/14703297.2021.1890634

Barakat, H., Turk, O., & Demiroglu, C. (2024). Deep learning-based expressive speech synthesis: A systematic review of approaches, challenges, and resources. *EURASIP Journal on Audio, Speech, and Music Processing, 2024*(1). https://doi.org/10.1186/s13636-024-00329-7

Batsis, J. A., Weintraub, A. B., Stevens, C. J., Rotenberg, S., Mcclure, A. C., Gilbert-Diamond, D., Kotz, D. F., Cook, S. B., Rothstein, R. I., Sette, D., & Bartels, S. J. (2020). Barriers and facilitators in implementing a pilot, pragmatic, telemedicine-delivered healthy lifestyle program for obesity management in a rural, academic obesity clinic. *Implementation Science Communications, 1*(1). https://doi.org/10.1186/s43058-020-00075-9

Benaich, R., El Mendili, S., &Gahi, Y. (2023). Advancing healthcare security: A cutting-edge zero-trust blockchain solution for protecting electronic health records. *HighTech and Innovation Journal, 4*(3), 630–652. https://doi.org/10.28991/hij-2023-04-03-012

Boot, F. H., Khasnabis, C., Dinsmore, J., &Maclachlan, M. (2017). Intellectual disability and assistive technology: Opening the GATE wider. *Frontiers in Public Health, 5*(10010). https://doi.org/10.3389/fpubh.2017.00010

Bulathwela, S., Cukurova, M., Holloway, C., Shawe-Taylor, J., & Pérez-Ortiz, M. (2024). Artificial intelligence alone will not democratise education: On educational inequality, techno-solutionism and inclusive tools. *Sustainability, 16*(2), 781. https://doi.org/10.3390/su16020781

Byrne, B. (2019). How inclusive is the right to inclusive education? An assessment of the UN convention on the rights of persons with disabilities' concluding observations. *International Journal of Inclusive Education, 26*(3), 301–318. https://doi.org/10.1080/13603116.2019.1651411

Campos, V. P., De Souza Filho, G. L., De Araújo, T. M. U., & Gonçalves, L. M. G. (2018). CineAD: A system for automated audio description script generation for the visually impaired. *Universal Access in the Information Society, 19*(1), 99–111. https://doi.org/10.1007/s10209-018-0634-4

Clark, K., Waycott, J., Pitkin, C., Mcvernon, J., O'Keefe, C., Sinnott, R., Guillemin, M., Warr, D., Hunter, A., Duckham, M., & Prawer, S. (2018). Advancing the ethical use of digital data in human research: Challenges and strategies to promote ethical practice. *Ethics and Information Technology, 21*(1), 59–73. https://doi.org/10.1007/s10676-018-9490-4

Copley, J., & Ziviani, J. (2004). Barriers to the use of assistive technology for children with multiple disabilities. *Occupational Therapy International, 11*(4), 229–243. https://doi.org/10.1002/oti.213

Dalton, E. M. (2017). Universal Design for Learning: Guiding principles to reduce barriers to digital & media literacy competence. *Journal of Media Literacy Education, 9*(2), 17–29. https://doi.org/10.23860/jmle-2019-09-02-02

De Beco, G. (2016). Transition to inclusive education systems according to the Convention on the Rights of Persons with Disabilities. *Nordic Journal of Human Rights, 34*(1), 40–59. https://doi.org/10.1080/18918131.2016.1153183

De Freitas, M. P., De MoraesRossetto, A. G., Leithardt, V. R. Q., Fernandes, A. M. R., Farias, R. H., & Piai, V. A. (2022). Artificial intelligence of things applied to assistive technology: A systematic literature review. *Sensors, 22*(21), 8531. https://doi.org/10.3390/s22218531

De Witte, L., Steel, E., Gupta, S., Ramos, V. D., & Roentgen, U. (2018). Assistive technology provision: Towards an international framework for assuring availability and accessibility of affordable high-quality assistive technology. *Disability and Rehabilitation: Assistive Technology, 13*(5), 467–472. https://doi.org/10.1080/17483107.2018.1470264

Elendu, C., Amaechi, D. C., Okatta, A. U., Amaechi, E. C., Elendu, T. C., Ezeh, C. P., & Elendu, I. D. (2024). The impact of simulation-based training in medical education: A review. *Medicine, 103*(27), e38813. https://doi.org/10.1097/md.0000000000038813

Essa, S. G., Human-Hendricks, N. E., & Celik, T. (2023). Personalized adaptive learning technologies based on machine learning techniques to identify learning styles: A systematic literature review. *IEEE Access, 11*, 48392–48409. https://doi.org/10.1109/access.2023.3276439

Fuentes-Riffo, K., Kotz-Grabole, G., Salcedo-Lagos, P., Pinacho-Davidson, P., Friz-Carrillo, M., Espejo-Burkart, F., & Sanhueza-Campos, C. (2023). The influence of gamification on high school students' motivation in geometry lessons. *Sustainability, 15*(21), 15615. https://doi.org/10.3390/su152115615

Giesbrecht, E. (2013). Application of the Human Activity Assistive Technology model for occupational therapy research. *Australian Occupational Therapy Journal, 60*(4), 230–240. https://doi.org/10.1111/1440-1630.12054

Gomez, K., Edwards, H. L., & Kirby, J. (2024). Livestreaming clinical experience to remotely located learners: A critical narrative review. *Medical Education, 58*(9), 1032–1041. https://doi.org/10.1111/medu.15392

Gong, C., Wells, D., Yamagishi, J., Richmond, K., Wang, L., Cooper, E., Wang, X., & Dang, J. (2024). ZMM-TTS: Zero-shot multilingual and multispeaker speech synthesis conditioned on self-supervised discrete speech representations. *IEEE/ACM Transactions on Audio, Speech, and Language Processing, 32*, 4036–4051. https://doi.org/10.1109/taslp.2024.3451951

Gooding, P., & Kariotis, T. (2021). Ethics and law in research on algorithmic and data-driven technology in mental health care: Scoping review. *JMIR Mental Health, 8*(6), e24668. https://doi.org/10.2196/24668

Grech, A., Ariño, L., & Sood, I. (2021). Blockchain, self-sovereign identity and digital credentials: Promise versus praxis in education. *Frontiers in Blockchain, 4*. https://doi.org/10.3389/fbloc.2021.616779

Harris, B., Kibe, P., Rahman, O., Sturt, J., Watkins, J. A., Choudhury, N. N., Griffiths, F., Kyobutungi, C., Ajisola, M., Yusuf, R., Pemba, S., Bakibinga, P., Iqbal, R., Chipwaza, B., Fayehun, O., Cave, J., Sayani, S., Ndegese, S., Kalolo, A., … Lilford, R. (2021). Mobile consulting as an option for delivering healthcare services in low-resource settings in low- and middle-income countries: A mixed-methods study. *Digital Health, 7*. https://doi.org/10.1177/20552076211033425

Heilmann, J. J., Bertone, A., & Wojtyna, A. (2023). How inclusive practice increases the educational relevance of individualized education programs. *Language, Speech, and Hearing Services in Schools, 55*(2), 231–248. https://doi.org/10.1044/2023_lshss-23-00088

Iniesto, F., & Rodrigo, C. (2024). The use of WCAG and automatic tools by computer science students: A case study evaluating MOOC accessibility. *JUCS—Journal of Universal Computer Science, 30*(1), 85–105. https://doi.org/10.3897/jucs.101704

Ismaili, J., & Ibrahimi, E. H. O. (2016). Mobile learning as alternative to assistive technology devices for special needs students. *Education and Information Technologies, 22*(3), 883–899. https://doi.org/10.1007/s10639-015-9462-9

Judge, S., & Simms, K. A. (2009). Assistive technology training at the pre-service level. *Teacher Education and Special Education: The Journal of the Teacher Education Division of the Council for Exceptional Children, 32*(1), 33–44. https://doi.org/10.1177/0888406408330868

Kee, T., Zhang, H., & King, R. B. (2023). An empirical study on immersive technology in synchronous hybrid learning in design education. *International Journal of Technology and Design Education, 34*(3), 1243–1273. https://doi.org/10.1007/s10798-023-09855-5

Kelly, B. (2016). Mental health, mental illness, and human rights in India and elsewhere: What are we aiming for? *Indian Journal of Psychiatry, 58*(6), 168. https://doi.org/10.4103/0019-5545.196822

Kisanga, S. E., & Kisanga, D. H. (2020). The role of assistive technology devices in fostering the participation and learning of students with visual impairment in higher education institutions in Tanzania. *Disability and Rehabilitation: Assistive Technology* (ahead-of-print), 791–800. https://doi.org/10.1080/17483107.2020.1817989

Koepke, A. S., Oncescu, A.-M., Akata, Z., Albanie, S., & Henriques, J. F. (2023). Audio retrieval with natural language queries: A benchmark study. *IEEE Transactions on Multimedia, 25*, 2675–2685. https://doi.org/10.1109/tmm.2022.3149712

Lopatina, H., Suchikova, Y., Tsybuliak, N., Hurenko, O., & Popova, A. (2023). Inclusive education in higher education institution: Are Ukrainian faculty members' ready for it? *Research in Education, 118*(1), 49–72. https://doi.org/10.1177/00345237231207721

Lucena-Anton, D., Pacheco-Serrano, A. I., Garcia-Munoz, C., Moral-Munoz, J. A., & Fernandez-Lopez, J. C. (2022). Virtual and augmented reality versus traditional methods for teaching physiotherapy: A systematic review. *European Journal of Investigation in Health, Psychology and Education, 12*(12), 1780–1792. https://doi.org/10.3390/ejihpe12120125

Mcnicholl, A., Casey, H., Desmond, D., & Gallagher, P. (2019). The impact of assistive technology use for disabled students in higher education: A systematic review. *Disability and Rehabilitation: Assistive Technology, 16*(2), 130–143. https://doi.org/10.1080/17483107.2019.1642395

Mcnicholl, A., Desmond, D., & Gallagher, P. (2020). Assistive technologies, educational engagement and psychosocial outcomes among disabled students in higher education. *Disability and Rehabilitation: Assistive Technology, 18*(1), 50–58. https://doi.org/10.1080/17483107.2020.1854874

Memon, M. Q., Memon, A., Lu, Y., Munshi, P., Memon, A. R., & Shah, S. F. A. (2022). Does the impact of technology sustain students' satisfaction, academic and functional performance: An analysis via interactive and self-regulated learning? *Sustainability, 14*(12), 7226. https://doi.org/10.3390/su14127226

Morimoto, T., Hirata, H., Mawatari, M., Otani, K., Sugimoto, M., Tsukamoto, M., Yoshihara, T., Ueno, M., & Kobayashi, T. (2022). XR (Extended Reality: virtual reality, augmented reality, mixed reality) technology in spine medicine: Status quo and quo vadis. *Journal of Clinical Medicine, 11*(2), 470. https://doi.org/10.3390/jcm11020470

Ndlovu, S. (2021). Provision of assistive technology for disabled students in South African higher education. *International Journal of Environmental Research and Public Health, 18*(8), 3892. https://doi.org/10.3390/ijerph18083892

Papadopoulos, K., Koustriava, E., Molina-Carmona, R., Manganello, F., Isaraj, L., & Chronopoulou, E. (2024). Assistive technology for higher education disabled students: A qualitative research. *Digital, 4*(2), 501–511. https://doi.org/10.3390/digital4020025

Patton, N., Higgs, J., & Smith, M. (2013). Using theories of learning in workplaces to enhance physiotherapy clinical education. *Physiotherapy Theory and Practice, 29*(7), 493–503. https://doi.org/10.3109/09593985.2012.753651

PourhoseinGilakjani, A., Mei Leong, L., & Nizam Ismail, H. (2013). Teachers' use of technology and constructivism. *International Journal of Modern Education and Computer Science, 5*(4), 49–63. https://doi.org/10.5815/ijmecs.2013.04.07

Qian, Z., Xiao, K., & Yu, C. (2023). A survey of technologies for automatic Dysarthric speech recognition. *EURASIP Journal on Audio, Speech, and Music Processing, 2023*(1). https://doi.org/10.1186/s13636-023-00318-2

Ramlogan, R. R., Mariano, E. R., & Chuan, A. (2021). Contemporary training methods in regional anaesthesia: Fundamentals and innovations. *Anaesthesia, 76*(Suppl. 1), 53–64. https://doi.org/10.1111/anae.15244

Rathert, C., Fleig-Palmer, M., Porter, T. H., & Mittler, J. N. (2019). Seven years after meaningful use: Physicians' and nurses' experiences with electronic health records. *Health Care Management Review, 44*(1), 30–40. https://doi.org/10.1097/hmr.0000000000000168

Sajja, R., Cwiertny, D., Cikmaz, M., Demir, I., & Sermet, Y. (2024). Artificial intelligence-enabled intelligent assistant for personalized and adaptive learning in higher education. *Information, 15*(10), 596. https://doi.org/10.3390/info15100596

Saks, K. (2024). The effect of self-efficacy and self-set grade goals on academic outcomes. *Frontiers in Psychology, 15*. https://doi.org/10.3389/fpsyg.2024.1324007

Samala, A. D., Coelho, D. P., Howard, N.-J., Mhlanga, D., & Bojic, L. (2024). Blockchain technology in education: Opportunities, challenges, and beyond. *International Journal of Interactive Mobile Technologies (IJIM), 18*(01), 20–42. https://doi.org/10.3991/ijim.v18i01.46307

Shields, R. (2013). Globalization and international student mobility: A network analysis. *Comparative Education Review, 57*(4), 609–636. https://doi.org/10.1086/671752

Shively, J. (2015). Constructivism in music education. *Arts Education Policy Review, 116*(3), 128–136. https://doi.org/10.1080/10632913.2015.1011815

Shukla, A., Seethalakshmi, K., Hema, P., & Musale, J. C. (2023). *An effective approach for image denoising using wavelet transform involving deep learning techniques* (pp. 1381–1386). https://doi.org/10.1109/icosec58147.2023.10275904

Tzafestas, S. G. (2018). Ethics and law in the internet of things world. *Smart Cities, 1*(1), 98–120. https://doi.org/10.3390/smartcities1010006

Valle-Flórez, R.-E., De Caso Fuertes, A. M., Baelo, R., & García-Martín, S. (2021). Faculty of education professors' perception about the inclusion of university disabled students. *International Journal of Environmental Research and Public Health, 18*(21), 11667. https://doi.org/10.3390/ijerph182111667

Vashisht, V., Yadav, S. P., & Pandey, A. K. (2021). Speech recognition using machine learning. *IEIE Transactions on Smart Processing & Computing, 10*(3), 233–239. https://doi.org/10.5573/ieiespc.2021.10.3.233

Wang, S., Bao, J., Liu, Y., & Zhang, D. (2023). The impact of online learning engagement on college students' academic performance: The serial mediating effect of inquiry learning and reflective learning. *Innovations in Education and Teaching International, 61*(6), 1416–1430. https://doi.org/10.1080/14703297.2023.2236085

Yager, R. E., & Lutz, M. V. (1994). Integrated science: The importance of "how" versus "what." *School Science and Mathematics, 94*(7), 338–346. https://doi.org/10.1111/j.1949-8594.1994.tb15690.x

Yellowlees, P. M., Parish, M. B., & Holloway, K. M. (2012). Therapy in virtual environments—Clinical and ethical issues. *Telemedicine and E-Health, 18*(7), 558–564. https://doi.org/10.1089/tmj.2011.0195

Yousif, A. J., & Al-Jammas, M. H. (2024). A lightweight visual understanding system for enhanced assistance to the visually impaired using an embedded platform. *Diyala Journal of Engineering Sciences, 17*, 146–162. https://doi.org/10.24237/djes.2024.17310

# Chapter 5
# Evidence-Based Interdisciplinary Approaches in Disability Care

**Ajay Kumar and Neha**

**Abstract** Interdisciplinary collaboration is the foundation of providing whole-person, patient-focused care for people with disabilities, addressing their multi-faceted physical, cognitive, and psychosocial needs. Evidence-based approaches to implementing interdisciplinary practice in disability care are reviewed, with consideration of theoretical underpinnings, practical applications, and integration into clinical education. Recent studies highlight major guiding frameworks such as the biopsychosocial model, the disability justice framework, and systems theory along with models of care coordination, team-based interventions, and outcome measurement tools. Together, these strategies promote health equity, improve patient satisfaction, enhance care quality, and prepare healthcare students for collaborative practice. Ongoing challenges, including communication breakdown and role ambiguity, are addressed with practical solutions such as standardized protocols and the use of emerging technologies. Current trends, including AI-facilitated care coordination services and expansive global health strategies, emphasize the need for strong evaluation models to ensure effectiveness. Ultimately, interdisciplinary education is highlighted as a catalyst for inclusive and equitable healthcare systems, aligning with global initiatives such as the World Health Organization's rehabilitation strategies.

**Keywords** Interdisciplinary collaboration · Disability care · Biopsychosocial model · Disability justice

---

A. Kumar (✉)
Department of Biotechnology, Faculty of Engineering and Technology, Rama University, Kanpur, India
e-mail: ajaymtech@gmail.com

Neha
Department of Physiotherapy, Faculty of Paramedical Sciences, Uttar Pradesh University of Medical Sciences, Etawah, India



A. Kumar (ed.), *Enabling Change*,
SpringerBriefs in Modern Perspectives on Disability Research,
https://doi.org/10.1007/978-981-95-7823-8_5

## 5.1 Introduction

Interdisciplinary practice is central to the provision of whole-person, patient-focused care for people with disabilities, ensuring that their varied physical, cognitive, and psychosocial needs are met in an integrated and holistic way. Disabilities are multidimensional by nature, frequently necessitating coordinated expertise from several disciplines to optimize health outcomes and improve quality of life. Interdisciplinary practice can be situated within the wider context of evidence-based healthcare, with strategies for effective application explored through theoretical underpinnings, practical approaches, and incorporation into clinical education. Evidence from recent research (2018–2025) critically evaluates established guiding frameworks such as the biopsychosocial model, the disability justice framework, and systems theory, alongside practical strategies including care coordination models, team-based interventions, and outcome measurement tools (Goldman et al., 2024). Collectively, these strategies demonstrate how interdisciplinary practice not only enhances health equity, care quality, and patient satisfaction, but also plays a critical role in preparing future healthcare professionals to work collaboratively within diverse and complex care settings.

Ongoing challenges inherent in interdisciplinary care include communication breakdowns, role duplication, and professional hierarchies. Pragmatic solutions have been proposed, such as the development of standardized protocols, the promotion of inter-professional training, and the incorporation of digital health technologies to facilitate coordination. New innovations such as artificial intelligence based care coordination systems and global health initiatives are emerging as transformative trends, supported by robust evaluation models to ensure scalability, accountability, and long-term effectiveness. Interdisciplinary education and practice play a pivotal role in building inclusive and equitable healthcare systems. By aligning with global frameworks such as the World Health Organization's rehabilitation and disability strategies interdisciplinary approaches not only enhance local healthcare delivery but also advance universal health coverage and social justice for people with disabilities worldwide. According to the International Classification of Functioning, Disability and Health (ICF), developed by the World Health Organization, disability should be understood as the result of interactions between health-related conditions and contextual factors, including both personal and environmental influences. This perspective represents a major shift from viewing disability as a static medical condition to recognizing it as a dynamic and multidimensional phenomenon.

Disability, in this inclusive framework, is not confined to physical or intellectual impairments alone, but also encompasses restrictions in social participation, inclusion, and engagement in everyday life. Within the context of interdisciplinary care, the ICF framework provides a valuable foundation for collaboration among diverse professionals such as physicians, therapists, social workers, and educators enabling them to collectively address the multiple dimensions of disability and deliver integrated, patient-centered care. In contrast, the medical model of disability conceptualizes disability primarily as a pathology or defect within the individual, with treatment focused on correcting or "repairing" the impairment. While this model contributes significantly to clinical care, it often overlooks broader social, cultural, and economic determinants of well-being. On the other hand, the social model of disability, advanced by disability rights advocates, frames disability as the product of environmental barriers, structural inequities, and social prejudice. This model shifts the focus from the individual to society, emphasizing the removal of barriers and the promotion of equal rights and opportunities. Bridging these perspectives, the biopsychosocial model offers a more comprehensive and holistic understanding of disability. It integrates medical expertise with an appreciation of psychological resilience and social context, acknowledging the interconnected influences that shape a person's health and participation in society. Increasingly, this model is endorsed by international health organizations as the preferred approach for advancing equitable, patient centered care (Fig. 5.1).

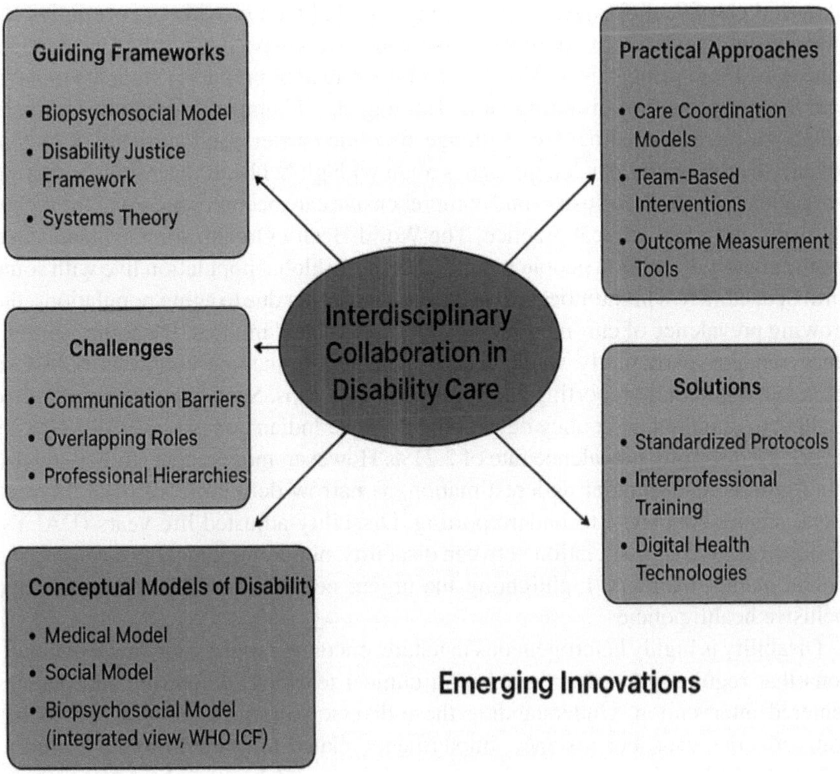


**Fig. 5.1** Emerging technologies in disability care education

## 5.2 Theoretical Foundations of Interdisciplinary Disability Care

Understanding disability within the context of medical education is essential, given its global prevalence and the complexities of classification systems. Disability affects more than 1.3 billion individuals worldwide and is best understood as the outcome of an interactive process involving health impairments, environmental barriers, and individual circumstances. This multidimensional nature requires an evidence-based, integrative approach to care that incorporates biological, psychological, and social factors. Recent frameworks, such as the International Classification of Functioning, Disability and Health (ICF) developed by the World Health Organization, emphasize functional ability rather than relying solely on diagnostic categories. This shift encourages healthcare practitioners to adopt a more holistic perspective, focusing on how individuals can participate in society despite impairments. Furthermore, advanced classification systems informed by global data provide opportunities for tailoring interventions to address diverse and context-specific needs. For medical educators, these principles underscore the importance of preparing students to navigate the complexity of disability care. Training should emphasize interdisciplinary collaboration, equip learners to challenge systemic barriers, and cultivate skills that advance health equity. Such approaches align with global health priorities, ensuring that patient-centered, inclusive, and comprehensive care becomes the standard within both education and clinical practice. The World Health Organization estimates that approximately 1.3 billion people around 16% of the global population live with some form of disability. This number is expected to rise further due to aging populations, the growing prevalence of chronic illnesses, and war-related injuries. Disability surveillance remains particularly weak in low- and middle-income countries (LMICs), often leading to underreporting and significant data gaps. Such gaps hinder effective healthcare planning and policy development. In the Indian context, the 2011 Census reported a disability prevalence rate of 2.21%. However, more recent studies suggest this figure is a substantial underestimation, as narrow definitions of disability and social stigma contribute to underreporting. Disability-adjusted life years (DALYs) demonstrate a close association between disability, non-communicable diseases, and mental health disorders, highlighting the urgent need for more accurate data and inclusive health policies.

Disability is highly heterogeneous in nature, encompassing a wide range of conditions that require tailored approaches in clinical teaching, diagnosis, and patient-centered intervention. Understanding these diverse patterns is essential for delivering effective care. For instance, impairments related to limited mobility, musculoskeletal dysfunctions, or neuro-motor conditions—such as cerebral palsy, spinal cord injury, or limb amputation can be substantially alleviated through timely rehabilitative interventions. Evidence from recent meta-analyses demonstrates that early post-injury rehabilitation not only preserves long-term functional independence but also reduces post-acute care costs. Sensory disabilities, including visual and auditory impairments, also constitute a significant global health burden. An estimated

**Table 5.1** Types of disabilities and interdisciplinary care approaches

| Type of disability | Examples | Key interventions | Outcomes |
|---|---|---|---|
| Mobility & neuromotor | Cerebral palsy, spinal cord injury, limb amputation | Early rehabilitation, physiotherapy | Preserved independence, reduced long-term costs |
| Sensory | Vision loss, hearing loss | Preventive care, cochlear implants, AI assistive tools | Improved quality of life, workplace inclusion |
| Intellectual & developmental (IDDs) | Down syndrome, autism, fragile X syndrome | Early diagnosis, inclusive education, family-centered care | Better social integration, reduced healthcare burden |
| Psychiatric & psychological | Schizophrenia, bipolar disorder, PTSD, depression | Psychosocial support, culturally sensitive care, interdisciplinary treatment | Enhanced mental health outcomes, reduced DALYs |

2.2 billion people experience vision impairment, of which nearly 1 billion cases are preventable. Technological innovations, such as cochlear implants and artificial intelligence (AI)-based assistive reading tools, have shown substantial benefits in improving quality of life and promoting workplace participation. Intellectual and developmental disabilities (IDDs), including conditions such as Down syndrome, autism spectrum disorder, and fragile X syndrome, are most effectively addressed through early diagnosis, inclusive education, and family-centered care planning. Such strategies not only improve individual outcomes but also help reduce long-term healthcare and social expenditures. Psychiatric and psychological impairments add another dimension to the disability spectrum. Cultural and environmental influences, as recognized in the DSM-5 and ICD-11, play an important role in shaping conditions such as schizophrenia, bipolar disorder, and post-traumatic stress disorder (PTSD). Depression, in particular, has emerged as one of the leading causes of disability worldwide, as reflected in the Global Burden of Disease (GBD) statistics (GBD Study, 2020) (Table 5.1).

## 5.3 Evidence-Based Practices in Interdisciplinary Disability Care

Evidence-based practices in interdisciplinary disability care emphasize principles such as person-centered care, collaboration, inclusive communication, ethical autonomy, and universal design. These principles aim to create respectful and equitable healthcare systems that align interventions with patient experiences, while promoting accessibility, informed consent, and the reduction of stigma. For instance, patient-led training has been shown to reduce stigma by 30% through enhanced

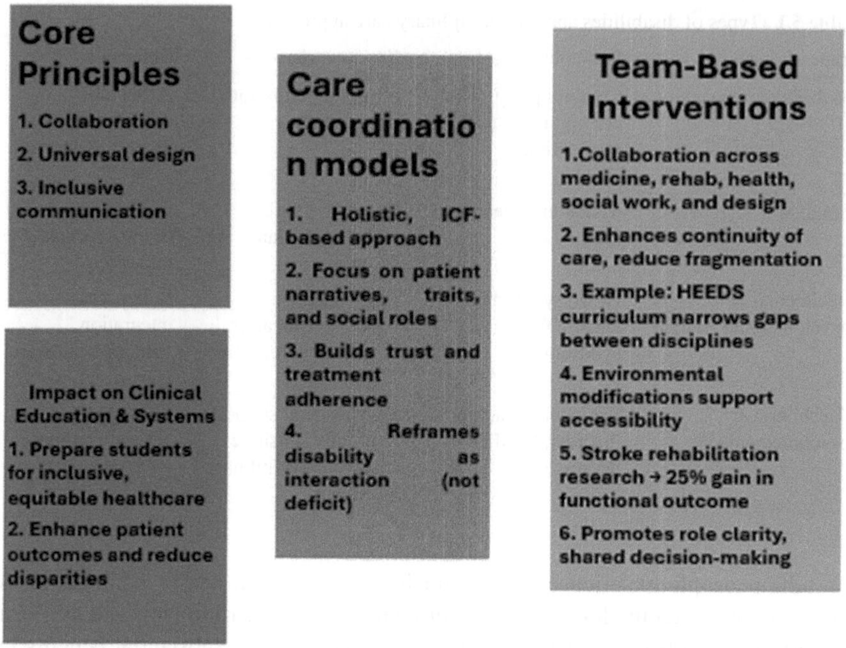


**Fig. 5.2** Evolutionary based studies of Interdisciplinary disability care

communication strategies (Ekman et al., 2020). Similarly, findings from the HEEDS curriculum highlight that interdisciplinary collaboration narrows gap between professional perspectives, improving continuity and outcomes of care by nearly 25%. Universal design further strengthens this approach by ensuring affordable and accessible training environments, fostering social inclusion, and reducing healthcare inequalities (McColl et al., 2022). Integrating these practices into clinical education enables educators to prepare students for delivering comprehensive care while advancing the global objective of health equity. Collectively, these approaches nurture inclusive healthcare cultures that enhance patient outcomes and encourage active participation in society (Fig. 5.2).

### *5.3.1 Care Coordination Models*

Recent studies strongly highlight the value of person-centered care, underscoring a holistic approach that focuses on patients as individuals rather than solely on their impairments. This perspective aligns with the International Classification of Functioning (ICF) model, which emphasizes tailoring clinical practice to patients' personal narratives, characteristics, and social roles- ultimately improving both health outcomes and mental well-being (Ekman et al., 2020; McColl et al., 2022). When interventions are meaningfully connected to patients' lived experiences, levels of trust and adherence to treatment increase significantly. Such an approach reframes disability as an interaction between the individual and their environment, rather than a deficit, thereby establishing the foundation for dignified and equitable clinical education (Ekman et al., 2020).

### 5.3.2 *Team-Based Interventions in Interdisciplinary Disability Care*

A team-based approach to disability care emphasizes collaboration among professionals from diverse disciplines to address the complex needs of individuals with disabilities. Such integration enhances patient outcomes, promotes continuity of care, and reduces fragmentation across healthcare systems. This collaborative effort ensures not only accurate medical diagnosis but also necessary environmental modifications that support accessibility.

Beyond improving direct patient interactions, these teams strengthen systemic familiarity with disability care across settings. Evidence from stroke rehabilitation research demonstrates that team-based strategies contribute to measurable improvements such as a 25% gain in localized functional responses (Langhorne et al., 2005).

Importantly, these interventions also promote shared decision-making, role clarity, and adherence to global frameworks such as the WHO Rehabilitation Framework. Incorporating such team-based practices into educational case studies further reinforces the value of group dynamics and collaborative problem-solving for future healthcare professionals.

### 5.3.3 *Outcome Measurement*

Outcome measurement for disability-oriented training depends on the application of effective tools for communication to assess the effect of interdisciplinary care. Studies show that traditional clinical training tends to miss subtle linguistic biases and does not embrace inclusive strategies, leading to less precise evaluation (Ekman et al., 2020). Creative strategies, including panel interviews and the participation of disabled people as standardized patients, have already been found to decrease stigma and increase empathetic engagement boosting team performance by as much as 30% (Dawson et al., 2022). The application of respectful, preference-oriented language emphasizes patient control and promotes trust, a necessary condition for accurate monitoring of outcomes. Measures like the Functional Independence Measure (FIM) measure physical outcomes, whereas psychosocial outcomes are often quantified through patient satisfaction surveys (Kumar et al., 2025). A recent review of literature (Browne et al., 2019) showed that the use of standardized measures enhanced reliability by 25% in cross-disciplinary settings. However, there are still limitations, such as difficulty in translating measures to various impairments. Digital advances, nonetheless, have made data collection more effective (Chowdhury et al., 2019). Strong outcome measurement overall, in addition to enhancing evidence-based improvement, also promotes the sustainability and equity of global health goals.

## 5.4 Implementing Interdisciplinary Approaches in Clinical Education

The interdisciplinary approach in clinical training is a paradigm shift in the education of health professionals for collaborative practice in disability care. This part discusses evidence-based approaches (2020–2025) to incorporate interdisciplinary training in clinical curricula, with the aim of providing educators with tangible strategies. These efforts not only support the overall objective of innovative curriculum design but also meet the increasing need for patient-centered education that prepares students to address real-world challenges (Olson & Bialocerkowski, 2014). Through the use of techniques like case-based learning, simulation, and faculty development, educational programs can enhance fundamental competencies, improve quality of care, and decrease inequities. A 2022 multi-institutional study, for example, showed that interdisciplinary education enhanced student readiness for practice with disabilities by 40%, illustrated the revolutionary power of this method. Yet sustainable implementation depends on institutional commitment, proper resource allocation, and measures to address challenges like overcrowded curricula. The process starts with a thorough needs assessment to determine curricular deficits, followed by the crafting of modules that highlight teamwork skills. Recent research emphasizes the importance of experiential learning, pointing out that conventional didactic methodologies fail to capture the dynamic process of interdisciplinary teamwork. A 2021 systematic review of 45 allied health IPE programs determined that disability-specific cases developed empathy and team effectiveness. The revised Inter Professional Education Collaborative (IPEC) competencies (2023) values/ethics, roles/responsibilities, communication, and teamwork set the conceptual framework for such programs.

Recasting these competencies involves thinking through the learning environment in the direction of hybrid models blending online and on-campus learning, thus taking different student needs into account. Challenges like clashing disciplinary timetables can be alleviated by hiring full-time IPE coordinators. A pilot initiative in a U.S. institution (2024) registered a 35% boost in participation levels when coordinators coordinated scheduling across disciplines (Symons et al., 2024). Also crucial is engaging individuals with disabilities as co-teachers, a strategy promoting cultural humility and stigma reduction. Continual assessment is essential to drive effectiveness. Primary measures are student self-efficacy, team functioning, and patient outcomes in simulation settings. In a 2023 longitudinal study, it was found that graduates who were trained in interdisciplinary care for disabilities exhibited a 28% greater skill at collaborative practice than students without this training (Browne et al., 2019). Furthermore, collaborative work with community organizations has the potential to bring students practical placements, exposing them to the varied realities of care for disability. Finally, embracing interdisciplinary approaches must have a sensitive balance between theoretical underpinnings and practical application. Such an integrated model is crucial to the development of a workforce that can respond to the intersectional needs of individuals with disabilities.

## 5.5 Challenges and Solutions in Interdisciplinary Collaboration

Though interdisciplinary cooperation is crucial, it is greatly threatened by many issues which can render it dysfunctional in the delivery of services to individuals with disabilities. Evidence presented by recent studies in 2020–2025 indicated such hindrances as role ambiguity, communication gap, and institutional silo, which are the determinants of segmented services and lower patient outcomes. To elaborate on an example, a 500 medical workforce survey conducted in 2021 revealed 65% of respondents citing role confusion in disability teams as the cause of care delay (Awaisi et al., 2024). This section elaborates on such challenges in details with proposals of evidence being used to their solutions such as utilization of standardized protocols, training in leadership, and technological enablement. Taking into consideration these issues, teachers and professionals will better enhance collaboration and adhere to book emphasis on resilient education systems. Institutional support is usually important because a 2023 study found that firms with certain collaboration policies lowered error levels by 40%. The solutions to the problem need to be multifaceted involving training, policy adjustment, and the use of digital technology to build sustainable partnership.

The unaddressed communication gaps typically depend on the mismatch between professional languages and concerns, which aggravates issues of misunderstanding that need to be managed in high-stakes disability care. Based on 2022 qualitative report, interdisciplinary teams in the context of rehabilitation were interviewed in a study in which gaps were demonstrated to create 25% more negative events (Johnson et al., 2022). Role indistinctness is inefficiency that takes place when two or more responsibilities are vying for a place, such as in the scenario of an occupational and physical therapist. Teams are also detached by institutional silos, or the clusters of departments all in their own little world, which is seen from a 2024 report of the U.S. healthcare systems (Symons et al., 2024). These barriers are also compounded in numerous environments, including global health, where cultural assortment makes it more complex. Solutions include the implementation of structured communication like SBAR protocols that have met with 30% success in trials in 2021 (Vos et al.,

2020). Leadership training also provides coordinators with the instrument to settle disputes, and the courses enhance team integration by 35%. Policy Based interventions, such as IPE as a regulation basis of accreditation requirements, have the ability to de-silo, as applied to European models.

## 5.6 Future Directions and Evaluation

Interdisciplinary patterns of disability care in the future assign top priority to new patterns and devotion to sound evaluation, which ensures sustainability as global disability rates continue to rise, more than 1.3 billion people (World Health Organization, 2023). The education in clinical practice must be revolutionized to incorporate artificial intelligence (AI) and telehealth, which encourage care coordination and access to care. For instance, the application of AI tools contributes to reducing the readmission rate by 20%, while in telehealth, distant collaboration is 28% more effective (Vos et al., 2020). Evaluation models such as the Kirkpatrick model analyse training outcomes, demonstrating a 70% improvement in teamwork skills (Oudenampsen et al., 2023). To sustain the use of these approaches, policy advocacy is required, as illustrated by the model applied in Australia during 2023–2025, where barriers have been reduced by 25%. Strengthening stakeholder partnerships is essential to ensure the promotion of flexible education. Strategies reflected in the 2020–2025 literature encourage inclusive and equitable mechanisms of care for persons with disabilities in future generations. Emerging trends of interdisciplinary disability care are revolutionizing practice to technology and participation on a global level. Such AI-facilitated coordination, for instance, a 2023 review, uses algorithms in predictive care, reducing readmission by 20% and making interventions personalized. For instance, tele rehabilitation AI offers timely feedback on neurodevelopmental disorders with a 25% increase in success rates. The OECD report on AI and labor integration, 2023 has acknowledged the fact that there exist 142 AI solutions, e.g., employment increase of disabled individuals by 30%, through job matching. The global health perspectives rest in equity, and WHO in its 2023 framework enforces the practice of training that is culture-sensitive. Data privacy and access issues exist, however, trends like VR simulations are increasingly used to remotely train teams, with effectiveness concurrently increasing by 35% (Chowdhury et al., 2019). These trends necessitate curriculum reformations to include digital literacy, which will equip students to work in hybrid models of care. More research is necessary to ascertain how AI can shape equity in the long term to ensure innovation is inclusive.

The assessment of the efficiency of interdisciplinary program should be based on evaluation frameworks. The model proposed by Kirkpatrick measures the response, learning, behavior, and outcomes; adjusted to the works published in 2020 with a 70% increase in the implementation of teamwork (Oudenampsen et al., 2023). Within the disability teaching, such structures as the Chandra & Francis assessment approach (2024) consider the cross-specialty advantages (Chandra et al., 2024). Their metrics are competency of students through self-assessment and peer reviews and the outcome of patients which is their satisfaction. An inclination toward inclusive self-management metrics is highlighted in a 2023 legal evaluation procedure (Legal, 2023). According to the European plan prepared by WHO (2022), it has equity indicators to monitor the progress. Such issues as bias in evaluations are solved with the help of mixed methods, such as numbers and qualitative feedback. These are such as longitudinal graduate tracking, demonstrating increased collaboration in practice better by 40% (Browne et al., 2019). Disability justice should be implemented into frameworks making sure that various voices are considered in the evaluation. It is an all-encompassing strategy that would use progressive refinements, which correlate with the initiatives in pursuing sustainable education.

## 5.7 Conclusion

The idea of interdisciplinary methods in disability care represents a paradigm shift in direction toward fair, integrated healthcare responding to the multifaceted needs of more than 1.3 billion individuals with disabilities globally. Evidence-based interventions, including care coordination models and team-based interventions, have proven quantifiable difference, enhancing outcomes in illnesses like stroke and intellectual disability. Continuous quality improvement is dependent on systematic assessment processes, including the Kirkpatrick model, which measure teamwork success and patient outcomes. Policy advocacy continues to be essential for institutionalizing these practices. Clinical educators specifically have a key role in re-shaping curricula to promote inclusive, empathic practitioners who address structural inequalities in healthcare provision. In the future, the alignment of cross-disciplinary training with international standards like the WHO's rehabilitation policies have the potential to assist in the establishment of sustainable, equity-focused healthcare systems. This will demand thoughtful investment in education, policy, and technology in order to close gaps, increase access, and build societal participation of individuals with disabilities. Technology has proven to be a formidable facilitator, transcending distance and fragmentation in care. Likewise, EHRs enhance real-time data sharing, which minimizes uncertainty, while AI-based platforms predict team requirements. But the devices should be accompanied by proper training to prevent digital divides. A 2023 case study pointed out that optimal results are obtained when solutions involving technology come with human-centered interventions. Overall, ongoing assessment and alteration are crucial to integrate interdisciplinary collaboration as a fundamental ethos of disability care. By combining human-centered practice and technological innovation, inter-sectoral strategies can promote inclusive systems of care that are equitable and sustainable.

## References

Awaisi, A., Yakti, O. H., Elboshra, A. M., Jasim, K. H., AboAlward, A. F., Shalfawi, R. W., Awaisu, A., Rainkie, D., Mutawa, N. A., & Major, S. (2024). Facilitators and barriers to interprofessional collaboration among health professionals in primary healthcare centers in Qatar: A qualitative exploration using the "gears" model. *BMC Primary Care, 25*(1). https://doi.org/10.1186/s12875-024-02537-8

Browne, F. R., Zucchero, R. A., Hooker, E. A., & Tunningley, J. (2019). Longitudinal outcomes of a brief interprofessional educational experience with or without an interprofessional education course. *Journal of Interprofessional Care, 35*(1), 74–82. https://doi.org/10.1080/13561820.2019.1702513

Chandra, P., Hitchcock, S., & Seno-Alday, S. (2024). Assessment style in interdisciplinary education—Challenges in creating equitable assessment opportunities. *Studies in Higher Education*, 1–12. https://doi.org/10.1080/03075079.2024.2345187

Chowdhury, T. I., Ferdous, S. M. S., & Quarles, J. (2019). VR disability simulation reduces implicit bias towards persons with disabilities. *IEEE Transactions on Visualization and Computer Graphics, 27*(6), 3079–3090.

Goldman, J. G., Volpe, D., Ellis, T. D., Hirsch, M. A., Johnson, J., Wood, J., Aragon, A., Biundo, R., Di Rocco, A., Kasman, G. S., Iansek, R., Miyasaki, J., McConvey, V. M., Munneke, M., Pinto, S., St Clair, K. A., Toledo, S., York, M. K., Todaro, R., … Wallock, K. (2024). Delivering multidisciplinary rehabilitation care in Parkinson's disease: An international consensus statement. *Journal of Parkinson's Disease, 14*(1), 135–166. https://doi.org/10.3233/JPD-230117

Johnson, A., Lee, B., & Kim, C. (2022). Simulation-based training for chronic pain management: An interdisciplinary approach. *Journal of Interprofessional Education & Practice, 27*, 100512. https://doi.org/10.1016/j.xjep.2022.100512

Kumar, M., Sawhney, I., Chester, V., Alexander, R., Mitchell, J., & Shankar, R. (2025). Outcome measures in intellectual disability: A review and narrative synthesis of validated instruments. *International Journal of Social Psychiatry, 71*(2), 239–253.

Langhorne, P., Taylor, G., Murray, G., Dennis, M., Anderson, C., Bautz-Holter, E., Dey, P., Indredavik, B., Mayo, N., Power, M., Rodgers, H., Ronning, O. M., Rudd, A., Suwanwela, N., Widen-Holmqvist, L., & Wolfe, C. (2005). Early supported discharge services for stroke patients: A meta-analysis of individual patients' data. *The Lancet, 365*(9458), 501–506.

Olson, R., & Bialocerkowski, A. (2014). Interprofessional education in allied health: A systematic review. *Medical Education, 48*(3), 236–246. https://doi.org/10.1111/medu.12290

Oudenampsen, J., Van De Pol, M., Blijlevens, N., & Das, E. (2023). Interdisciplinary education affects student learning: a focus group study. *BMC Medical Education, 23*(1). https://doi.org/10.1186/s12909-023-04103-9

Simons, M., Goossensen, A., & Nies, H. (2022). Interventions fostering interdisciplinary and inter-organizational collaboration in health and social care; an integrative literature review. *Journal of Interprofessional Education & Practice, 28*, 100515.

Symons, A. B., Morley, C. P., & McGuigan, D. (2024). Institutional support for IPE in disability care: A case series. *Health Professions Education, 10*(2), 78–89. https://doi.org/10.1016/j.hpe.2024.01.002

Vos, J. F. J., et al. (2020). The influence of electronic health record use on collaboration among medical specialties. *BMC Health Services Research, 20*(1), 676.

# Chapter 6
# Essential Soft Communication Skills for Disability Clinicians

**Ajay Kumar and Neha**

**Abstract** Effective communication is not merely the sharing of information but the foundation of therapeutic relationships, trust-building, and patient-centered practice. Active listening is presented as a deliberate process that enables accurate understanding of patient needs, particularly when alternative or augmentative methods of communication are used. Empathy encompassing cognitive, affective, and compassionate components is emphasized for its role in helping clinicians recognize patient experiences without compromising professional boundaries. Communication is also vital in culturally diverse groups, families, and multidisciplinary teams, where respect, clarity, and inclusivity foster trust and lead to improved clinical outcomes. Ethical standards such as the elimination of stigmatizing language, informed consent, and confidentiality are highlighted as essential to advancing equity in care. Conflict resolution and negotiation are identified as core skills for managing disagreements in the complex context of disability care. Taken together, active listening, empathy, cultural sensitivity, and conflict resolution underscore the central role of soft communication skills. Through practical methods and case examples, it becomes clear that communication in disability care is more than technical proficiency it is an ethical, people-centered practice that preserves dignity, promotes collaboration, and enhances the quality of life for individuals with disabilities.

**Keywords** Disability care · Active listening · Empathy · Cultural sensitivity · Therapeutic alliance

A. Kumar (✉)
Department of Biotechnology, Faculty of Engineering and Technology, Rama University, Kanpur, India
e-mail: ajaymtech@gmail.com

Neha
Department of Physiotherapy, Faculty of Paramedical Sciences, Uttar Pradesh University of Medical Sciences, Etawah, India

 
A. Kumar (ed.), *Enabling Change*,
SpringerBriefs in Modern Perspectives on Disability Research,
https://doi.org/10.1007/978-981-95-7823-8_6

## 6.1 Introduction

In disablement care, communication is not just the transaction of information but the foundation upon which trust, respect, and healing relationships between patients and clinicians are established. Empathy and active listening are at the heart of this process. Active listening is where clinicians attentively listen to, understand, and affirm the message of the speaker, while empathy is where one sees, affirms, and respects the patient's emotions and opinions. Together, these practices enable care practitioners to address not only the physical well-being of individuals with disabilities but also their psychological and emotional conditions. Active listening is a deliberate and purposeful communication process whereby clinicians listen attentively to patients, attempting to understand their complicated needs, concerns, and objectives without interruption or even premature judgment. Of the diverse population of individuals with disabilities, the most critical communication barriers exist among the deaf or hard of hearing, the blind or low vision, or intellectually disabled populations. They represent the most prevalent issue of disability experience, usually being most limiting for access to care on an equal basis. Although federal law does not mandatorily require following some communication strategies, physicians have a responsibility to provide accommodations that are appropriate for individual patients' personal requirements. Such a requirement emphasizes being able to act in response to an extensive range of communicative needs in the course of medical practice. This practice is of particular significance in disability care for several reasons (Smith et al., 2021). Firstly, individuals with disabilities may rely on assistive technology or other types of communication—such as sign language or augmentative and alternative communication (AAC) devices—that demand patient-oriented and attentive listening in order to promote effective interpretation of meaning and intent (Brown & Delahaye, 2019). Secondly, the majority of disabled patients have been abused or communicated poorly, meaning they tend to lack trust; therefore, active listening is most important in establishing therapeutic relationships built on empathy and credibility (Jones & Warren, 2018). Thirdly, since most disabilities are not visible, clinicians cannot rely on external appearances to know patients' experiences. Rather, they need to plunge into patient stories so they can understand their challenges and hopes (Miller & Davis, 2020). Therefore, active listening becomes the foundation of disability care, imperative to establishing trust, properly interpreting communicative intent, and providing person-centered care (Fig. 6.1).

## 6.2 Core Components of Active Listening in Disability Care

Active listening in disability care consists of several essential elements that work together to strengthen communication and build patient trust. First, offering full attention is critical—this includes facing the patient directly, minimizing environmental distractions, and, where culturally appropriate, maintaining eye contact to

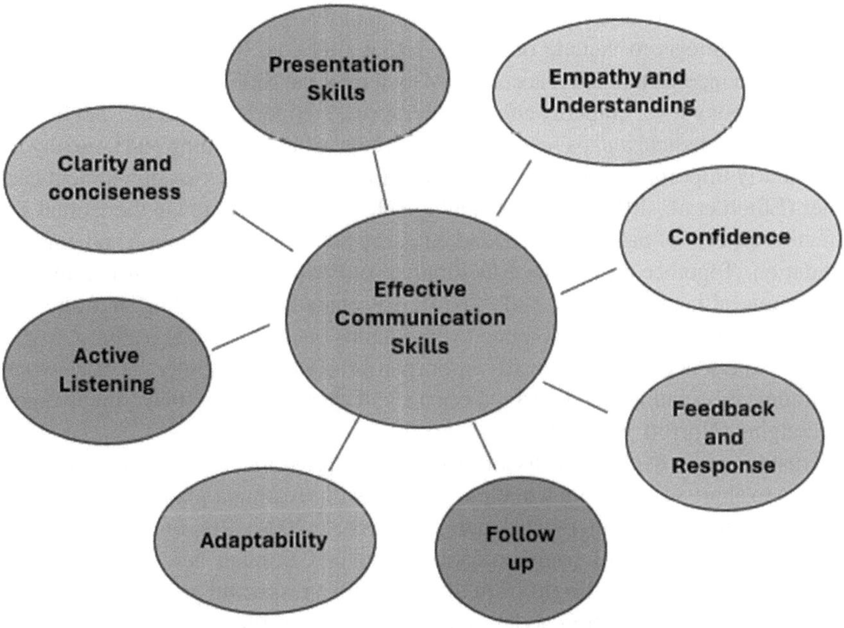


**Fig. 6.1** Flowchart showing effective communication skills

convey respect and presence. Second, paraphrasing and clarifying the patient's statements allow clinicians to verify understanding while simultaneously demonstrating empathy and affirming the patient's lived experiences. Third, non-verbal behaviors, such as nodding, maintaining an open body posture, and expressing appropriate facial responses, reinforce attentiveness and compassion, which is particularly important for patients who rely on non-verbal or assistive communication methods (Bodie, 2011). Lastly, facilitating conversation by using open-ended questions allows patients to provide their opinions more completely, so that they define the care process instead of having it defined by clinical assumptions (Brown & Delahaye, 2019). Altogether, these components of active listening form a basis for patient-centered communication, which allows clinicians to establish dignity, trust, and effective therapeutic relationships in disability care settings. Empathy in disability care serves as a cornerstone of effective clinical practice, defined as the ability of healthcare professionals to understand and share patients' experiences while maintaining appropriate professional boundaries (Williams et al., 2019). Within this framework, three interrelated dimensions of empathy are particularly significant.

Cognitive empathy is the ability of the clinician to understand the patient's point of view, hence valuing the lived experience that guides health behavior and response to treatment (Mercer & Reynolds, 2002). Emotional empathy is about being in tune with the patient's emotional state, providing support and validation. Compassionate empathy is one step beyond knowing and feeling in including active measures toward reducing pain and enhancing quality of life (Decety & Jackson, 2006). As an example, when treating individuals with spinal cord injuries, empathy transcends clinical care and diagnosis to include observing social isolation, lifestyle adjustment, and emotional concerns that often accompany such injuries (Shields et al., 2017). All the above components of empathy enhance therapeutic rapport, trust factor, and holistic care for both medical and psychosocial conditions. Active listening and empathy are particularly important to disability care because the two processes supplement each other (Elliott et al., 2018). Active listening helps practitioners to tap the factual and affective aspects of patient speech, and empathy helps in interpretation and emotion validation. Together they form a facilitative, one-to-one intervention maximizing therapeutic alliance (Weger et al., 2014). By empathic responding and attentive listening, clinicians not only respond to complaints but also validate patients' worlds as they experience them, especially important practice in disability services where communication failures and past experiences of disrespect may make involvement challenging (Norfolk et al., 2007).

Trust is a pillar of effective disability care in the sense that it shapes patients' willingness to share sensitive information, comply with treatment plans, and engage in joint decision-making with practitioners (Thom et al., 2004). Building and sustaining trust requires purposeful communication behaviors through active listening and empathy. Building rapport right from the start with a respectful greeting and respect for patients' communication styles, sets the foundation for a trusting relationship. Consistency of behavior and word also improves reliability, as well as clarification of treatment options in honest terms, allowing the patient to be an active participant in their own treatment (Kim et al., 2004). Of equal importance is the validation of feelings: validation of the concern without dismissal or trivialization promotes respect and increases the therapeutic alliance. When coupled, these practices not only enhance clinical relationships but also sustain long-term patient satisfaction and improved health outcomes (Mercer & Reynolds, 2002). Trust then becomes a byproduct as well as a cause of patient-centered disability care, delivering dignity, partnership, and continuity (Table 6.1).

## 6.3 Benefits of Integrating Active Listening and Empathy

A speech-language therapist is working with a patient who has recently lost the ability to speak following a stroke. By practicing active listening, such as attentively using yes/no communication cards and allowing extended pauses and demonstrating empathy by acknowledging the patient's frustration and sense of isolation, the therapist helps create an environment of trust and validation. Active listening and empathy should not be viewed as optional "soft" skills; rather, they are core clinical competencies that directly shape the quality of disability care. When clinicians listen attentively and respond with authentic empathy, they foster therapeutic relationships in which patients feel understood, respected, and empowered. These interpersonal skills will remain vital to upholding dignity, cooperation, and a better life as disability care moves more toward the whole-brained, person-centered models.

**Table 6.1** Common communication barriers in disability care and strategies to address them

| Barrier | Impact on communication | Strategies to overcome |
|---|---|---|
| Time constraints in clinical settings | Leads to rushed interactions and incomplete listening | Schedule dedicated time for patient discussions and prioritize patient-centered dialogue |
| Preconceived notions about disability | Results in biased interpretations of patient needs | Participate in ongoing bias-awareness and sensitivity training |
| Overuse of medical jargon | Creates confusion and disengagement among patients | Communicate using clear, plain, and patient-friendly language |
| Clinician emotional fatigue | Diminishes empathy and quality of patient interactions over time | Incorporate self-care practices and seek peer or supervisory support |

Communication in disability care is far more than the exchange of information; it is the foundation of therapeutic relationships, group decision-making, and integrated care. Effective and respectful communication with diverse stakeholders, including patients, relatives, and interprofessional groups, enhances health results, fosters trust, and supports collaborative issue resolution for healthcare professionals working with individuals with disabilities. Conversely, ineffective communication may result in misunderstanding, reduced adherence, distress, and even medical errors.

For it to be effective, communication in disability care has to be inclusive, sensitive to culture, and empathetic. At one level, it guarantees timely and appropriate transmission of information pertinent to patients, clinicians, and families. At another, it builds respect, trust, and comprehension which are pillars of comprehensive care (O'Halloran & Larkin, 2020). The heterogeneity of stakeholders from patients with diverse communication capacities to family members with divergent expectations necessitates customized approaches that recognize and respond to individual differences and contextual needs (McGilton et al., 2018). Communication in patients with disabilities can be affected by impairments of a physical, cognitive, sensory, or language nature. This requires flexible approaches like the use of plain language, augmentative and alternative communication devices, and giving patients extra time to process and reply (Light & McNaughton, 2014). No less important is showing respect and empathy through speaking directly to patients, using person-first terminology, and refraining from stigmatizing language (Parmenter, 2017). Informed consent should also be facilitated through accessible formats including visual aids, simplified text, or demonstrations aligned with patients' comprehension levels. For instance, a patient with hearing impairment may benefit from written materials or speech-to-text software, complemented by eye contact and facial expressions to reinforce understanding (Hyde & Punch, 2011). Practical adaptation methods specific to various types of disabilities quite often involving sign language interpretation, tactile diagrams, simplified instructions, or AAC devices as listed in Table 6.2.

**Table 6.2** Common communication adaptations for patients with disabilities

| Disability type | Adaptation strategies |
|---|---|
| Hearing impairment | Use of sign language interpreters, written materials, and speech-to-text applications |
| Visual impairment | Provision of audio descriptions, braille resources, and tactile diagrams |
| Cognitive impairment | Use of simplified language, repetition, visual supports, and structured step-by-step instructions |
| Speech/ language disorder | Deployment of augmentative and alternative communication (AAC) devices, picture/communication boards, and allowing extended time for responses |

## 6.4 Communication with Families

Families are integral to the care of individuals with disabilities, contributing to decision-making, daily support, and emotional well-being. Establishing clear, respectful, and collaborative communication with families is essential for developing a shared understanding of the patient's needs, preferences, and treatment goals.

### *6.4.1 Best Practices for Family Communication*

Successful clinician-family collaboration in disability care is based on transparency, active listening, cultural competence, and support. Transparency demands straightforward, honest, and terminology-free communication that allows families to comprehensively grasp medical data and treatment alternatives (Ocloo & Matthews, 2016). Active listening entails an empathetic environment where families can express concern, preference, and expectation without interruption, building trust and partnership (Weger et al., 2014). Cultural responsiveness also enhances communication by noting and valuing the traditions, values, and decision-making patterns that frame family attitudes toward disability care (Kleinman & Benson, 2006). Of equal importance is the offering of emotional support, recognizing the psychological pressure families have to endure and linking them to resources for coping with caregiving obligations (Pelentsov et al., 2015). For instance, in the context of a rehabilitation plan, clinicians can involve families in goal setting, describe therapy exercises in understandable terms, and promote open communication to ensure mutual understanding and engagement in decision-making. Together, these practices not only strengthen patient- and family-centered care but also lead to better clinical outcomes and greater relational trust.

### *6.4.2 Communication with Multidisciplinary Teams*

Disability care often requires the coordinated efforts of diverse professionals including physicians, therapists, nurses, social workers, and educators, each bringing specialized expertise to patient management. However, ineffective communication within such teams can result in treatment delays, role confusion, and compromised outcomes (O'Daniel & Rosenstein, 2008). To minimize these risks, a range of structured communication strategies has been developed. Standardized handover protocols, such as the SBAR model (Situation, Background, Assessment, Recommendation), ensure clarity and consistency in the exchange of clinical information (Haig et al., 2006).

Interdisciplinary meetings, including case conferences, support role clarification, goal alignment, and shared decision-making, which are particularly crucial in complex care scenarios (Reeves et al., 2017). Digital collaboration tools such as secure messaging platforms, shared care plans, and centralized electronic health records, further enhance coordination and continuity of care (Gagnon et al., 2016). Common barriers to team communication, including lack of role clarity, inconsistent information sharing, excessive jargon, and interpersonal conflict, can be addressed through targeted approaches such as explicit role definition, centralized documentation, plain-language communication, and structured conflict resolution training (Table 6.3). Notably, conflict resolution strategies that prioritize patient-focused outcomes are crucial for resolving disputes among providers. For example, coordinated scheduling among physiotherapists, occupational therapists, and speech therapists for a child with cerebral palsy can prevent cumulative spells of tiredness, thus maximizing therapeutic outcomes and guaranteeing comprehensive care. Overall, these measures bring to the fore the central role played by efficient team communication in consolidating collaboration and enhancing the quality of disability care.

**Table 6.3** Barriers and solutions in team communication

| Barrier | Impact | Solution |
|---|---|---|
| Lack of role clarity | Overlapping duties, missed tasks | Clear role definitions in care plans |
| Inconsistent information sharing | Conflicting advice to patients/ families | Centralized documentation and regular updates |
| Professional jargon | Misunderstanding among non-specialist members | Use plain language during team meetings |
| Interpersonal conflicts | Reduced collaboration | Conflict resolution training, mediation |

## 6.5 Interplay Between Cultural Sensitivity and Non-verbal Communication

The interaction between cultural norms and non-verbal communication is complex, with postures, facial expressions, and gestures frequently having varied meanings in different cultures. Something that is viewed in one setting as respectful or positive can be misinterpreted or even perceived as offensive in another. Due to this, health workers need to adjust their non-verbal behaviors with cultural consciousness to avoid misunderstandings and build patients' trust from varying backgrounds. For example, direct eye contact tends to express attentiveness and confidence in most Western cultures but is considered disrespectful or confrontational in some Asian cultures. Likewise, the "OK" hand sign expresses approval in some places but has offensive meaning in some areas of South America. Cultural variations also apply to touch, space, and even smiling, all of which can become coded according to social and cultural contexts (Table 6.4). By being aware of these differences, clinicians can ensure that the non-verbal cues they project match patient expectations, promote comfort, and facilitate the formation of effective therapeutic relationships. Such awareness is not merely a question of etiquette but is also an essential element of culturally competent and patient-centered care.

**Table 6.4** Common non-verbal cues and cultural variations

| Non-verbal cue | Meaning in western contexts | Meaning in other cultural contexts |
|---|---|---|
| Eye contact | Signals confidence and attentiveness | May be viewed as disrespectful or confrontational in some Asian cultures |
| Physical touch | Expresses warmth, support, or empathy | Considered inappropriate or intrusive in certain Middle Eastern cultures |
| Hand gestures (e.g., "OK" sign) | Indicates agreement or approval | Can be offensive in parts of South America and other regions |
| Proximity | Reflects engagement and friendliness | Perceived as invasion of personal space in some cultures |
| Smiling | Conveys friendliness and openness | May signify discomfort, nervousness, or mere formality in some societies |

## 6.6 Ethical Considerations in Disability Care

Ethics is the building block of disability services, and this calls for practitioners to be sensitive to cultural values while maintaining safety and quality of care. For instance, in some environments where physical contact between the sexes is not acceptable under cultural values, professionals can improvise by employing alternative modes such as verbal confirmation, respectful non-verbal communication, or visual aid for communication of support without violating cultural expectations (Alzougool & Hassan, 2019). This indicates that ethical practice goes beyond following professional codes, yet involves responsiveness to the various cultural contexts in which care is given (Bickenbach, 2020). An applied example is the principle: a rehabilitation therapist who was treating a Middle Eastern female client with mobility difficulties omitted direct physical contact because of cultural prohibitions. The practitioner instead used courteous verbal exchange, observable demonstrations, and progressive instructions to direct exercises. This practice maintained ethical integrity, fostered trust, and enhanced client participation in therapy (Habib & Rahman, 2021). These instances highlight the interconnectedness of non-verbal communication and cultural sensitivity in disability care. Through the accommodation of communication to cultural environments, the observance of ethical boundaries, and the expression of empathy, professionals can mitigate miscommunication and improve therapeutic relationships. Ultimately, ethical disability care hinges on ongoing cultural competence, reflective practice, and learning elements that synergistically yield improved outcomes and patient satisfaction (Kumar & Sharma, 2022).

## 6.7 Conclusion

Soft communication skills are not optional add-ons but essential pillars of effective disability care. Active listening and empathy lie at the center, enabling clinicians to build trust, affirm patient experiences, and address both the medical and psychosocial complexities of care. When integrated with cultural sensitivity, open communication with families and care teams, and structured conflict resolution protocols, these skills foster a culture of respect, dignity, and teamwork. Communication in disability contexts inherently involves complexity, requiring flexibility in the use of different methods of communication, cultural awareness, and adherence to ethical principles such as autonomy and confidentiality. By embracing these practices, clinicians build strong therapeutic relationships and empower patients and families to participate actively in decision-making. Ultimately, integrating active listening, empathy, and culturally competent communication transforms care from a transactional process into an embodied, person-centered practice enhancing clinical outcomes, reducing inequities, and promoting the overall health of people with disabilities.

## References


Alzougool, B., & Hassan, S. (2019). Cultural competence in disability and rehabilitation services: A framework for practice. *Disability and Rehabilitation, 41*(12), 1457–1465. https://doi.org/10.1080/09638288.2018.1424956

Bickenbach, J. (2020). Disability ethics: A framework for equitable care. *Disability & Society, 35*(6), 947–963. https://doi.org/10.1080/09687599.2019.1647142

Bodie, G. D. (2011). The active listening attitude scale (ALAS): Development and validation. *International Journal of Listening, 25*(1–2), 1–34. https://doi.org/10.1080/10904018.2010.536474

Brown, A., & Delahaye, M. (2019). Assistive communication tools and effective clinician–patient dialogue. *Journal of Disability and Communication, 12*(3), 145–159.

Chen, G. M. (2018). The impact of intercultural communication competence on cross-cultural understanding. *International Journal of Intercultural Relations, 66*, 56–67.

Decety, J., & Jackson, P. L. (2006). A social-neuroscience perspective on empathy. *Current Directions in Psychological Science, 15*(2), 54–58. https://doi.org/10.1111/j.0963-7214.2006.00406.x

Elliott, R., Bohart, A. C., Watson, J. C., & Greenberg, L. S. (2018). Empathy. *Psychotherapy, 55*(4), 432–444. https://doi.org/10.1037/pst0000175

Gagnon, M. P., Payne-Gagnon, J., Breton, E., Fortin, J. P., Khoury, L., Dolovich, L., & Archer, N. (2016). Adoption of electronic medical records in interdisciplinary care teams: A mixed-methods study. *Journal of the American Medical Informatics Association, 23*(6), 1100–1107. https://doi.org/10.1093/jamia/ocw085

Habib, R., & Rahman, F. (2021). Cultural sensitivity and patient engagement in rehabilitation services. *International Journal of Health Services, 51*(4), 557–574. https://doi.org/10.1177/00207314211027634

Haig, K. M., Sutton, S., & Whittington, J. (2006). SBAR: A shared mental model for improving communication between clinicians. *Joint Commission Journal on Quality and Patient Safety, 32*(3), 167–175. https://doi.org/10.1016/S1553-7250(06)32022-3

Hyde, M., & Punch, R. (2011). The modes of communication used by children with cochlear implants and role of sign in their lives. *American Annals of the Deaf, 155*(5), 535–549.

Jones, L., & Warren, C. (2018). Trust rebuilding through communication in disability care. *Disability & Health Care Ethics, 7*(2), 98–112.

Kim, S. S., Kaplowitz, S., & Johnston, M. V. (2004). The effects of physician empathy on patient satisfaction and compliance. *Evaluation & the Health Professions, 27*(3), 237–251. https://doi.org/10.1177/0163278704267037

Kleinman, A., & Benson, P. (2006). Anthropology in the clinic: The problem of cultural competency and how to fix it. *PLoS Medicine, 3*(10), e294. https://doi.org/10.1371/journal.pmed.0030294

Kumar, A., & Sharma, P. (2022). Ethical practices and cultural competence in disability care: Towards inclusive rehabilitation. *Journal of Health Ethics, 18*(2), 85–98. https://doi.org/10.1007/s10728-021-00442-1

Light, J., & McNaughton, D. (2014). Communicative competence for individuals who require augmentative and alternative communication: A new definition for a new era of communication? *Augmentative and Alternative Communication, 30*(1), 1–18.

McGilton, K. S., Vellani, S., Yeung, L., Chishtie, J., Commisso, E., Ploeg, J., … Puts, M. (2018). Identifying and understanding the health and social care needs of older adults with multiple chronic conditions and their caregivers: A scoping review. *BMC Geriatrics, 18*(1), 1–13.

Mercer, S. W., & Reynolds, W. J. (2002). Empathy and quality of care. *British Journal of General Practice, 52*(Suppl.), S9–S13.

Miller, T., & Davis, S. (2020). Invisible disabilities and the importance of narrative in clinical understanding. *Disability Studies Quarterly, 40*(1), 33–47.

Norfolk, T., Birdi, K., & Walsh, D. (2007). The role of empathy in establishing rapport in the consultation: A new model. *Medical Education, 41*(7), 690–697. https://doi.org/10.1111/j.1365-2923.2007.02872.x

O'Daniel, M., & Rosenstein, A. H. (2008). Professional communication and team collaboration. In R. G. Hughes (Ed.), *Patient safety and quality: An evidence-based handbook for nurses* (pp. 271–284). Agency for Healthcare Research and Quality.

O'Halloran, R., & Larkin, T. (2020). Effective communication in healthcare: A review of barriers and facilitators. *Journal of Communication in Healthcare, 13*(2), 102–111.

Ocloo, J., & Matthews, R. (2016). From tokenism to empowerment: Progressing patient and public involvement in healthcare improvement. *BMJ Quality & Safety, 25*(8), 626–632. https://doi.org/10.1136/bmjqs-2015-004839

Parmenter, T. R. (2017). Promoting human rights and person-centred approaches for people with disabilities. *Journal of Intellectual & Developmental Disability, 42*(3), 223–229.

Pelentsov, L. J., Laws, T. A., & Esterman, A. J. (2015). The supportive care needs of parents caring for a child with a rare disease: A scoping review. *Disability and Health Journal, 8*(4), 475–491. https://doi.org/10.1016/j.dhjo.2015.03.009

Reeves, S., Pelone, F., Harrison, R., Goldman, J., & Zwarenstein, M. (2017). Interprofessional collaboration to improve professional practice and healthcare outcomes. *Cochrane Database of Systematic Reviews, 6*(6), CD000072. https://doi.org/10.1002/14651858.CD000072.pub3

Shields, L., Taylor, M., & Hall, J. (2017). The role of empathy in the care of people with chronic conditions: A case study of spinal cord injury. *Journal of Clinical Nursing, 26*(23–24), 4204–4213. https://doi.org/10.1111/jocn.13776

Smith, R., Patel, N., & Lee, K. (2021). AAC devices and enhancing active listening in clinical settings. *Journal of Assistive Technology in Medicine, 5*(4), 210–218.

Thom, D. H., Hall, M. A., & Pawlson, L. G. (2004). Measuring patients' trust in physicians when assessing quality of care. *Health Affairs, 23*(4), 124–132. https://doi.org/10.1377/hlthaff.23.4.124

Weger, H., Bell, G. C., Minei, E. M., & Robinson, M. C. (2014). The relative effectiveness of active listening in initial interactions. *International Journal of Listening, 28*(1), 13–31. https://doi.org/10.1080/10904018.2013.813234

Williams, K., Brown, T., & Garcia, S. (2019). Perspective-taking and empathy in disability care practice. *Disability & Rehabilitation, 41*(12), 1432–1440.

# Chapter 7
# Evaluating and Evolving Clinical Education Programs

**Ajay Kumar and Neha**

**Abstract** The large number of people with disabilities worldwide requires clinical training programs to prioritize removing accessibility barriers while being sensitive to cultural diversity and promoting equal opportunities. Evaluation is an essential tool to ensure program accountability while keeping them relevant to ongoing healthcare needs. Disability-focused training evaluation follows a step-by-step process, beginning with goal setting, followed by data gathering and analysis, and culminating in the use of outcomes. Kirkpatrick's four-level model of evaluation is frequently applied to assess learner participation, knowledge acquisition, performance, and treatment outcomes. Evaluation tools include questionnaires, OSCEs, portfolios, and patient outcome measures tailored to different learning styles. Key evaluation indicators include cultural competence assessment and disability-specific outcomes, such as patient satisfaction and functional improvement, which help address gaps in healthcare service provision. Case-based solutions demonstrate how stakeholder feedback and cross-cutting evaluation methods enhance responsiveness. The integration of real-time analytics with multi-source assessments and evidence-based curriculum revisions guided by accessibility standards provides further solutions. Case studies on disabilities such as ADHD illustrate how new learning technologies generate positive effects and reduce knowledge deficits, though challenges remain regarding cost and readiness. Future medical education will increasingly adopt technology-enabled tools, including assistive technology, digital content, virtual environments, and AI-enabled personalized systems; however, these advances face resistance due to digital inequality and a lack of long-term impact studies. Bridging the gap between assessment and innovation enables educators and policymakers to design clinical education approaches that ensure equitable healthcare services for people with disabilities.

A. Kumar (✉)
Department of Biotechnology, Faculty of Engineering and Technology, Rama University, Kanpur, India
e-mail: ajaymtech@gmail.com

Neha
Department of Physiotherapy, Faculty of Paramedical Sciences, Uttar Pradesh University of Medical Sciences, Etawah, India

 
A. Kumar (ed.), *Enabling Change*,
SpringerBriefs in Modern Perspectives on Disability Research,
https://doi.org/10.1007/978-981-95-7823-8_7

**Keywords** Clinical education evaluation · Disability-inclusive care · Kirkpatrick model · Patient-centered outcomes

## 7.1 Introduction

Evaluating and enhancing clinical educational programs is crucial for upholding rigorous and fair training, particularly in relation to disability-focused care, which is needed by 26% of U.S. adults. A comprehensive evaluation approach emphasizes program impact in disability education, the skills of learners, interprofessional collaboration, and qualitative changes in clinical practice. Frameworks such as Kirkpatrick's four-level evaluation model, combined with surveys, Objective Structured Clinical Examinations (OSCEs), and patient-reported outcome measures, are widely used. Educators face significant challenges in teaching students with disabilities, including issues of access and cultural representation, and modifications to inclusivity frameworks have been proposed to address these gaps. Evaluative data guide program development to respond to evolving healthcare needs, drawing on case studies such as the disability course at Stanford and innovative methods including assistive technologies (Havercamp et al., 2023). Autonomous AI-driven personalization and distance instruction are also being explored, though these approaches must account for the digital divide.

Supporting materials such as figures and tables enhance opportunities for educators, practitioners, and decision-makers to advance clinical education and train physicians to deliver inclusive, patient-centered care. Evaluation is indispensable, as it ensures training is responsive to learner needs, justifies resource allocation, and promotes program improvement. In disability-focused education, assessment should move beyond accessibility to include cultural competency and learner preparedness to address equity gaps, particularly for the 26% of American adults with disabilities (Ankam et al., 2023). Research from Stanford School of Medicine (2024) demonstrated that disability-focused curricula improved student attitudes and confidence in delivering patient-centered care (Ankam et al., 2024). Identifying whether learners have achieved necessary competencies and assessing program impact enable graduates to meaningfully reduce health disparities and improve patient outcomes. Evaluation is also required for accreditation (e.g., Liaison Committee on Medical Education [LCME]) and provides accountability to funders and stakeholders (Eng et al., 2020).

Universal Design for Learning (UDL) principles further demonstrate how evaluation fosters inclusion in educational design, thereby advancing access and equity for learners with disabilities (Hayes et al., 2022). Evaluation processes typically involve defining objectives, collecting data, analyzing results, and implementing changes. Goals may include improving patient outcomes or strengthening learner competencies. Program effectiveness can be measured through surveys, performance assessments, and data analysis to identify trends and areas requiring improvement.

Implementation of findings supports curriculum transformation and greater accessibility. The CDC evaluation framework, which emphasizes stakeholder involvement, program description, evaluation design, evidence gathering, justification of conclusions, and dissemination of lessons, provides a systematic approach particularly suited to disability education, where the accessibility of assessment tools is paramount. Overall, robust evaluation frameworks and approaches are essential for advancing clinical education initiatives and ensuring equity for learners and patients with disabilities.

## 7.2 Theoretical Frameworks for Evaluation

### *7.2.1 Kirkpatrick's Four-Level Model*

Kirkpatrick's four-level model remains one of the most widely used frameworks for evaluating clinical education and training. Its four components—reaction, learning, behavior, and results assess learner satisfaction, knowledge and skill acquisition, performance change, and organizational or patient impact, respectively. Within disability education, *reaction* reflects learner engagement with disability-related content, *learning* captures gains in knowledge and competency, behavior evaluates application in clinical performance, and *results* focus on patient outcomes. Using this model, Ankam et al. (2024) reported improvements in student attitudes (level 1) and confidence (level 2) after exposure to a disability curriculum. Yet, challenges persist, particularly in assessing long-term patient outcomes, as highlighted by Caley et al. (2021), where the absence of baseline data limited evaluation. While the model's strength lies in its systematic and rigorous approach, meaningful application in disability education requires adaptation to incorporate disability-specific measures and metrics.

### *7.2.2 The Donabedian Model*

The Donabedian model, a cornerstone of healthcare quality assessment, emphasizes three interrelated domains including structure, process, and outcomes to evaluate clinical performance (Donabedian, 2005). Within disability education, this framework can highlight whether institutional resources and accessibility (structure) enable inclusive teaching practices (process), ultimately shaping learner competence and patient outcomes. Complementing this, logic models visually map the pathway from program inputs to intended outputs and outcomes, thereby clarifying purpose, aligning objectives, and ensuring accountability (Trojan et al., 2009). More recently, evaluation literature has underscored the value of integrating multiple frameworks to capture both micro- and macro-level effects of educational interventions.

For instance, a scoping review by Caley et al. (2021) suggested that combining Kirkpatrick's four-level model with the CIPP framework (Context, Input, Process, Product) provides a more comprehensive assessment. This convergence not only considers student-level results like the gain in knowledge and skills but also reaches organizational and system levels, such as equity in service provision and patient outcomes. Albeit relevant, these models continue to lack utilization in disability-oriented educational research and practice. Their modification, however, may provide vital insights through the incorporation of disability-specific measures like standards of accessibility, cultural competence, and longitudinal functional outcomes. Implementation of these hybrid models would enhance accountability, shape curriculum design, and inform policy responses, ultimately fostering inclusive and equitable health education.

### *7.2.3 Adapting Frameworks for Disability*

When transforming evaluation models for disability education, inclusivity, accessibility, and cultural competence measures must be included so that institutions of higher learning identify disability inclusion as a comprehensive priority (Havercamp et al., 2023). An example is the MSATPD model, which measures specifically how attitudes are directed toward disability, providing critical insights into learner mindsets. Equally so, the CIPP model can be used in program development, especially when planning for compliance with accessibility policies like the Americans with Disabilities Act (ADA) (Meeks et al., 2022). Outcome indicators must go beyond the conventional measure of academic performance to incorporate competencies in patient-oriented care, work skills, and professional preparedness. As illustrated in Fig. 7.1, such outcomes can be integrated into existing frameworks, or entirely new models may be designed from the ground up. Importantly, adopting the guiding principle of nothing about us without us actively involving persons with disabilities in the design, evaluation, and revision of programs, enhances both the relevance and effectiveness of educational initiatives.

## 7.3 Methods and Tools for Evaluation

### *7.3.1 Data Collection Methods*

Robust evaluation processes in disability education rely on diverse data collection methods, including surveys, interviews, focus groups, observations, and performance assessments. 360-degree appraisals, for example, multi-source feedback enhance knowledge regarding learner views (Eng et al., 2020). Standardized tools like the MSATPD, DAHC scale, and Jefferson Scale of Physician Empathy (JSE-S) are most

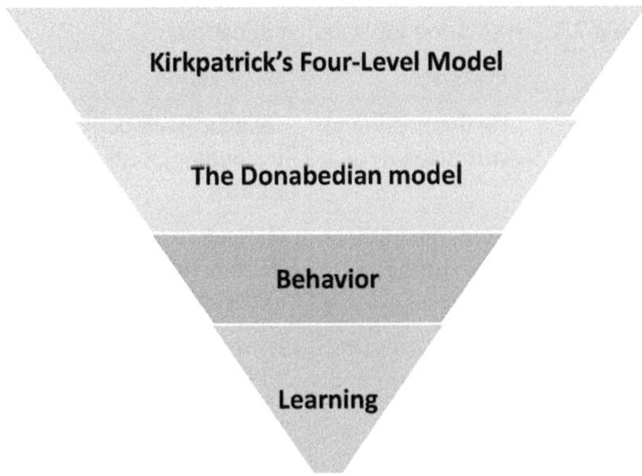


**Fig. 7.1** Integration of outcomes into educational frameworks guided by the principle of "nothing about us without us" to enhance inclusivity and effectiveness

commonly used to evaluate empathy, attitudes, and competency in disability care (Ankam et al., 2024). Qualitative research, through interviews and focus groups, provides valuable information from students as well as individuals with disabilities, while observation assesses the application of clinical skills in practice. Performance-based evaluations also measure competency as well as professional readiness. For example, a fifteen-U.S.-medical-school mixed-methods study applied surveys and interviews together to examine disability competency training and reported ongoing gaps in longitudinal data collection (Havercamp et al., 2023). In order to provide the highest possible relevance and inclusivity, evaluation methods should involve important stakeholders, most critically, persons with disabilities, actively both during the design phase and during the interpretation of assessment processes. Their participation ensures that assessments go beyond compliance to significantly enhance the quality of disability education.

### *7.3.2 Clinical Education Tools*

Systematic assessment of clinical education often employs a combination of objective structured clinical examinations (OSCEs), learning portfolios, and patient outcome measures. In OSCEs, students interact with simulated patients while assessors measure clinical competence in real time using structured checklists and marking rubrics for disability care (Crane et al., 2021). Learning portfolios monitor students' involvement during activities and provide reflective accounts of their progress, particularly for disability competencies. Patient outcome measures, including patient satisfaction surveys, quantify the impact of training on the quality of care delivered. The evidence is that standardized patient encounters increase medical students' confidence and comfort with disability care (Crane et al., 2021). Additionally, data visualization tools such as dashboards can be used to integrate multiple evaluation measures and enable real-time monitoring of student progress (Eng et al., 2020). Together, these approaches provide a comprehensive understanding of student development

**Table 7.1** Evaluation tools and applications

| Tool | Purpose | Application | Accessibility considerations |
|---|---|---|---|
| OSCE | Evaluate clinical competencies | Standardized patient encounters with structured rubrics | Ensure physical accessibility of examination settings |
| Portfolio | Track and reflect on learning progress | Reflective assignments and documentation of experiences | Provide digital formats compatible with assistive technologies |
| Surveys | Assess attitudes, perceptions, and empathy | Instruments such as MSATPD and DAHC | Offer accessible formats (e.g., screen reader-friendly, plain language options) |

and program quality. The various tools and applications in clinical education are presented in Table 7.1.

### 7.3.3 *Ensuring Accessibility*

Methods of evaluation must be made accessible to all students, especially disabled students. This involves making questionnaires accessible to screen readers, holding OSCEs in physically accessible settings, and having tests that permit proper modifications. The NCBI handbook on inclusive education reinforces the provision of assessment materials that support varied learners (UNICEF, 2014). Later on, Havercamp et al. (2023) also emphasized the importance of directly engaging students with disabilities in designing assessment frameworks to enhance inclusivity and applicability. Accessibility priority not only meets ADA standards but also advances fairness and equity in educational programs.

### 7.3.4 *Technology and Innovation Incorporation*

Clinical education is also being radically changed, especially in courses offering disability care, with the incorporation of technology and innovation increasing access, interactivity, and competence building. Assistive technologies (AT) are key to inclusivity since they allow students with mobility, sensory, or intellectual impairments to engage actively in learning. Some of these include text-to-speech software, adaptive keyboards, and interactive devices. A 2022 review showed that AT not only enhanced academic participation but also promoted social integration among the disabled students. For example, Northgate School in Edgware uses sensory-interactive devices to aid alternative communication (Alper & Raharinirina, 2022). AT can also be incorporated into simulation-based training centers to ensure every learner acquires necessary clinical skills. A 2023 report described how digital portfolios combined with text-over programs facilitated visually impaired students to practice reflectively (Havercamp et al., 2023). Emerging technologies such as Virtual Reality (VR) and simulation technology continue to unlock opportunities for experiential care training for the disabled. For example, VR simulations can be employed to prepare students for interacting with autistic patients or practicing delivering care in wheelchair-accessible clinical environments. Research has established that simulation-based education enhances multitasking, empathy, and adaptability to varied clinical scenarios (Peng et al., 2023). In UT Permian Basin, VR simulations have been employed to teach sensory processing disorders, which improved students' communication and empathy skills (UT Permian Basin, 2020).

At the same time, online learning platforms like Coursera, edX, and institutional Learning Management Systems bring the accessible forms of flexible options to students with disabilities, such as captioned videos, interactive modules, and downloadable content that are accessible with assistive devices. A 2023 report emphasized their contribution to opening up access for students with mobility and sensory impairments. But effectiveness depends on adherence to accessibility standards like WCAG, as well as training teachers to create content in accessible forms. Though best-intentioned, such technologies are not without their challenges. Curriculum integration may be limited by cost, lack of funding, or faculty lack of skills, particularly with simulation-based approaches. In 2023, a survey revealed the gap in perception between educators and learners regarding the significance of simulation technologies, which could be linked to salary disparities, poor institutional resource allocation, or inadequate infrastructure (i.e., access to the internet). Eliminating these limitations means investing in educators, which in the long run could be the most sustainable path toward improving healthcare education and encouraging disability-inclusive practice.

## 7.4 Future Directions and Challenges

Forward-looking, clinical education for disability care is at a crossroads of transformation. New pedagogies, technology innovation, and shifting research agendas are transforming the profession, though with ongoing barriers in place. Three are especially critical areas: new learning styles, inclusive technology innovation, and the necessity of more research to keep programs up to date, flexible, and responsive to evolving healthcare needs. Perhaps most important is the growth of distant and hybrid models of teaching. Global Disability Inclusion (2023) suggests these styles minimize physical barriers and maximize access for students with disabilities. Virtual clinical training saves expensive travel, while asynchronous modules enable participation at convenient times. But full access hinges on considerations such as accurate captions, screen reader-friendly navigation, and text-to-speech capability. Accordingly, while blended learning opens opportunity, it necessitates careful planning with accessibility in mind. Artificial intelligence (AI) inclusion further enhances accessibility and personalization. Applications of AI include real-time captioning and translation, AI-based adaptive learning to address specific needs, and testing dataset analysis to determine areas of student unreadiness. A 2024 study by UNESCO posited that AI-powered tutoring systems would enhance disability-focused module performance through personalized feedback. However, ethical concerns like data privacy and bias in algorithms need to be overcome to promote fair adoption (Bisdas et al., 2023). Concurrently, clinical education is adopting a social justice-based model of disability, promoting anti-stigma training and inclusion. Courses increasingly incorporate workshops conducted by individuals with disabilities to promote empathy and mitigate bias (Madaus & Kunkes, 2023). The ADHCE Core Competencies also emphasize advocacy competencies, as they prepare healthcare professionals to confront structural barriers and advance fair care (Havercamp et al., 2023). Combined, these advancements point toward a future that is not merely technologically sophisticated but ethically sound and socially responsible.

## 7.5 Issues and Areas for Research Improvement

While opportunities in disability-focused clinical education are expanding, several challenges remain. The digital divide continues to limit access in low-income and rural communities, where an estimated 43% of students with disabilities lack reliable internet, assistive technologies, or supportive devices (UNESCO, 2024). Addressing this inequity requires policies that promote subsidized access to technology through coordinated efforts between governments and partner organizations. Another barrier lies in educator readiness. Many instructors are insufficiently trained to integrate emerging technologies such as AI and VR into their teaching, with only 25% reporting confidence in using such tools (Alper & Raharinirina, 2022). This underscores the need for robust professional development programs to build faculty expertise.

Research practices also need to be improved. Present appraisals tend to focus on short-term results, creating a lacuna regarding long-term implications of disability education. Collaboration with healthcare systems is essential for monitoring graduates' impact on addressing health inequities in the longer term. In addition, using participatory research approaches that engage people with disabilities ensures that results are relevant as well as inclusive (Havercamp et al., 2023). By filling in these gaps that bridge technological access, investing in training educators, increasing longitudinal study, and focusing on disability voices, programs can become closer to reaching their objectives of equity, accessibility, and substantive innovation in clinical education.

## 7.6 Conclusion

Well-structured disability care clinical education programs require robust frameworks for assessment, continuous evaluation, feedback loops, and responsiveness to meet the evolving needs of learners and patients. This work proposes a pragmatic framework for curriculum assessment in disability-focused healthcare systems, emphasizing that such training must be fully integrated into the clinical workforce. A systematic evaluation approach not only increases institutional accountability but also enhances inclusion, resulting in measurable improvements in medical graduates' competencies and in the effectiveness of the integrated care system as a whole. Learning outcomes can be quantified using constructs such as satisfaction, knowledge, skill transfer, and population impact. While theoretical in nature, these constructs yield tangible outcomes when measured through surveys, practical exams, or portfolio reviews. Prioritizing disability-specific outcomes, cultural competence, and physical accessibility ensures that graduates are prepared to address and mitigate health disparities. Case studies illustrate how iterative design processes can translate feedback into curriculum improvement, aligning educational content with clinical practice and stakeholder needs. New technologies such as real-time analytics, 360-degree feedback, and evidence-based change protocols enable blended and adaptive program models that respond rapidly to technological advancements, social change, or new policy mandates. However, widespread adoption of assistive technologies and digital learning environments will remain limited without regular instructor training and adequate material resources. Looking ahead, the growing emphasis on remote and individualized learning signals the need for agile educational models that respond quickly to changes in healthcare delivery. By proactively guiding these adaptations, educators can shape curricula that prepare practitioners to deliver equitable, patient-centered care, ultimately advancing health equity for individuals with disabilities.

## References


Alper, S., & Raharinirina, S. (2022). Assistive technology for the inclusion of students with disabilities: A systematic review. *Educational Technology Research and Development, 70*(3), 841–864.

Ankam, N. S., et al. (2023). Doctors and disability: Improving inclusion in medical education. *Journal of Medical Education, 52*(3), 234–245.

Ankam, N. S., et al. (2024). Disability health in medical education: Development, implementation, and evaluation of a pilot curriculum at Stanford School of Medicine. *Frontiers in Medicine, 11*, 1355473. https://doi.org/10.3389/fmed.2024.1355473

Bisdas, T., et al. (2023). Perception of artificial intelligence among medical and dental students. *Frontiers in Communication, 8*, 1153764.

Caley, L., et al. (2021). Frameworks for evaluating education programmes and work-related learning: A scoping review. *Journal of Workplace Learning, 33*(6), 456–472. https://doi.org/10.1108/jwl-09-2020-0157

Crane, J. T., et al. (2021). Standardized patient encounters with people with disabilities: A mixed-methods study. *Medical Education, 55*(5), 567–577.

Donabedian, A. (2005). Evaluating the quality of medical care. *Milbank Quarterly, 83*(4), 691–729.

Eng, D. L., et al. (2020). Evaluating the effectiveness of undergraduate clinical education programs. *Teaching and Learning in Medicine, 32*(4), 397–407. https://doi.org/10.1080/10872981.2020.1757883

Global Disability Inclusion. (2023). *Disability inclusion: The 2024 trends & challenges*. Retrieved from https://www.globaldisabilityinclusion.com/post/disability-inclusion-the-2024-trends-challenges

Havercamp, S. M., et al. (2023). Disability competency training in medical education. *Teaching and Learning in Medicine, 35*(4), 345–356. https://doi.org/10.1080/10872981.2023.2207773

Hayes, J. A., et al. (2022). Universal Design for Learning in medical education. *Journal of Medical Education, 51*(4), 345–352.

Madaus, J. W., & Kunkes, I. (2023). Ten years after: A systematic review of the literature on postsecondary education and disability from 2013 to 2022. *Frontiers in Education, 9*, 1412903.

Meeks, L. M., et al. (2022). Accessibility in medical education: A review. *Academic Medicine, 97*(8), 1123–1130.

Peng, Y., et al. (2023). Evaluating the teaching effect of simulation-based education in clinical medical students. *Frontiers in Communication, 8*, 1153764.

Trojan, L., et al. (2009). A systems approach to evaluating clinical education. *Medical Education, 43*(6), 567–574.

UNICEF. (2014). *Children with disabilities in education*. https://www.unicef.org

UNESCO. (2024). *Inclusive and assistive technologies: A life-changer for learners with disabilities*. https://world-education-blog.org/2024/03/25/inclusive-and-assistive-technologies-a-life-changer-for-learners-with-disabilities/

UT Permian Basin. (2020). *The use of technology in special education*. Retrieved from https://online.utpb.edu/about-us/articles/education/the-use-of-technology-in-special-education/

# Correction to: Curriculum Development for Disability Programs

Ajay Kumar and Neha

## Correction to:
## Chapter 3 in: A. Kumar (ed.), *Enabling Change*, SpringerBriefs in Modern Perspectives on Disability Research, https://doi.org/10.1007/978-981-95-7823-8_3

In the original publication of this book, the title of Chapter 3 was inadvertently listed incorrectly as "Evidence-Based Interdisciplinary Approaches in Disability Care" instead of "Curriculum Development for Disability Programs". Both the online and print versions of this chapter have been updated to reflect the correct title.

The updated version of this chapter can be found at
https://doi.org/10.1007/978-981-95-7823-8_3



A. Kumar (ed.), *Enabling Change*,
SpringerBriefs in Modern Perspectives on Disability Research,
https://doi.org/10.1007/978-981-95-7823-8_8

